Autism Antidotes:

Unveiling the ASD causes and Management

By

Joseph E. Torres

Table of contents

Introduction

Conclusion

Introduction

What is Autism?

Autism, also known as autism spectrum disorder (ASD), is a complex condition characterized by difficulties with behavior and communication. It may involve numerous symptoms and abilities. ASD can be a minor issue or a disability that necessitates 24-hour care in a specialized facility. Autism patients struggle with communication. They struggle to comprehend other people's thoughts and feelings. Because of this, it's hard for them to express themselves verbally or through touch, facial expressions, and gestures. Learning difficulties may arise in people with autism. Their abilities could grow unevenly. They might, for instance, have difficulty communicating but be exceptionally adept at math, art, music, or memory. They might do particularly well on tests of analysis or problem-solving because of this.

Today, more children than ever before are diagnosed with autism. However, the most recent figures may not reflect an increase in the number of children with the disorder; rather, they may reflect changes in how it is diagnosed.

A neurological and developmental disorder known as autism spectrum disorder (ASD) affects how people interact with others, communicate, learn, and behave. Autism is known as a "developmental disorder" because symptoms typically begin in the first two years of life, despite the fact that it can be diagnosed at any age.

The American Psychiatric Association's Diagnostic and Statistical Manual of Mental Disorders (DSM-5), which medical professionals use to diagnose mental disorders, states that people with ASD frequently exhibit the following characteristics:

Autism is referred to as a "spectrum" disorder due to the wide range of symptoms experienced by individuals with the condition. These symptoms include difficulty communicating with others and engaging in social interactions, restricted interests, and repetitive behaviors.

ASD can be diagnosed in people of any gender, race, ethnicity, or economic status. Treatments and services for ASD can improve a person's symptoms and daily functioning, even though the disorder can last a lifetime. All children should be tested for autism, as the American Academy of Pediatrics advises. A screening or evaluation for ASD should be discussed with the child's doctor.

ASD signs and symptoms The following is a list of some typical behaviors that people with ASD are found to exhibit. The majority of people with ASD will exhibit several of the following behaviors, though not all of them.

Examples of social interaction and communication behaviors include: Not responding or being slow to respond to one's name or to other verbal bids for attention Having difficulties with the back and forth of conversation Frequently talking at length about a favorite subject without noticing that others are not interested or without giving others a chance to respond Displaying facial expressions, movements, and gestures that do not match what is being said Having an uncommon

tone of voice that may sound monotonous or flat and machine-like
Having issues understanding another person's perspective or being unable to
Having a persistent, intense interest in particular subjects, such as numbers, details, or facts. Displaying much focused interests, such as with objects in motion or portions of objects. Getting upset by small changes in routine and having trouble transitioning. Being more detective or less detective than other people to sensory input, such as light, sound, clothing, or temperature. Individuals with ASD may also be exposed to sleep disorder and peevishness.

Additionally, people on the autism spectrum may possess numerous strengths, such as:

Being able to learn in detail and remember information for a long time. Being a strong visual and auditory learner. Being an expert in math, science, music, or art.

What does being unique feel like?

The Cherokee tribe and the Native of Americans had a well recognized proverb saying that "you should never judge an individual before you have gone a mile in their shoes". It's practical advice to see a circumstance from the point of view of another before giving an opinion. One can observe how this type of thought can lead to a great level of compassion and understanding of people around us.

But how can an individual really experience the point of view of another?

It's certainly easier said than done. Consider the case of individuals with autism. These days almost every individual has heard of the word autism or autism spectrum disorders (ASD), both generalized terms for a group of complex and unusual occurrences of brain development. These disorders are classified, in varieties of degrees, by difficulties in social interaction, verbal and nonverbal interactions and possible repetition of behaviors. Hence, according to the research of the Centers for Disease Control (CDC), the current incidence of autism is 1 out of 68 children.

A lack of ability to process all of a person's environment's sensory inputs is one of the main symptoms of autism. People on the spectrum frequently exhibit hypersensitivity to sights and sounds. In most cases, this causes stress and anxiety to rise. As a means of coping with the mental chaos they are experiencing, an autistic person may make "unnatural gestures" like swinging their arms, rocking back and forth, or other movements.

It is essential to be able to replicate this experience for people who are neurotypical because sensory overload, anxiety, and confusion that accompany it, are essential components of comprehending autism.

Chapter one:
Diagnosis, signs/symptoms and types of Autism

Diagnosis:

Children with autism spectrum disorder (ASD) and their families can benefit greatly from early diagnosis.

However, it is not always simple to diagnose ASD. Doctors rely on observing the behaviors of very young children and listening to their parents' concerns because there is no lab test for it.

The symptoms of ASD range widely. Mental impairments can be severe in some "on the spectrum" individuals. Others are capable of self-sufficiency and high intelligence.

Getting an autism diagnosis for your child, regardless of where they fall on the spectrum, is a two-step process that begins with your pediatrician.

Well-Child Visits Pediatricians are the first person to diagnose an individual with autism. Even if a child does not appear to have any symptoms, they are assessed at their 18- and 24-month checkups to ensure that they are on track.

Your child's pediatrician will observe and interact with them at these appointments. They will inquire about your child's development and behavior, family history, and whether anyone in the family has autism. Your doctor will be looking for a few key points:

At six months, did your infant smile?

By nine months, did they imitate sounds and facial expressions?

By the time they were 12 months old, were they babbling and cooing?

They'll also inquire about the following:

or recurring?

Is it something difficult for them to coincidentally make eye contact?

Do they talk to others and share their experiences?

When someone tries to get their attention, do they respond?

Does their voice seem "flat"?

Do they comprehend what other people do?

Are they sensitive to temperature, noise, or light?

Are you having trouble sleeping or digesting?

Are they typically irritated or irate?

Your responses are very important to the screening of your child.

That's the end of it if nothing goes wrong and you have no concerns.

However, your doctor will refer you to a specialist for additional tests if your child exhibits developmental issues or if they have concerns.

Additional Tests Your child's next appointment probably will be with a team of ASD specialists, including a child psychologist, speech-language pathologist, and occupational therapist, if your child needs additional tests. Additionally, you may meet with a neurologist and a developmental pediatrician.

Your child's cognitive level, language skills, and other life skills like eating, dressing, and using the bathroom are typically checked during this evaluation.

Your child must meet the requirements of the Diagnostic and Statistical Manual of Mental Disorders (DSM-5) published by the American Psychiatric Association in order to receive an official diagnosis.

For your child to be on the autism spectrum, he or she must have issues in two areas.

1. Difficulties with social interaction and communication. Reading social cues, making eye contact, having a conversation, and "connecting" with other people are difficult for children with ASD. It's possible that they won't speak as soon as other children do. Additionally, they might struggle with the muscle skills required for activities like sports or writing and drawing.

2. patterns of behavior that are restricted and consistent. Changes in routine can cause ASD children to rock their bodies, repeat words, or become upset. They frequently have a strong interest in a single topic. Additionally, they have sensory issues.

A new device that utilizes data and artificial intelligence to assist in the diagnosis of ASD may be used by your child's doctor if they exhibit potential symptoms of the disorder. The Cognoa ASD Diagnosis Aid is software based on machine learning that monitors children aged 18 months to 5 years and assists in assessing and determining any developmental issues. Early diagnosis and treatment can be crucial to your child's development of useful skills.

Genetic testing may also be recommended by your child's doctors to rule out any other conditions that could cause these symptoms.

Signs/Symptoms of Autism:

What signs and symptoms does ASD have?

The following is a list of some typical behaviors that people with ASD exhibit. The majority of people with ASD will exhibit several of the following behaviors, though not all of them.

Examples of social interaction and communication behaviors include: 'Making little or inconsistent eye contact' 'Appearing not to look at or listen to people who are taking' 'Infrequently sharing interest, emotion, or enjoyment of objects or activities (including infrequently pointing at or showing things to others)' 'Having difficulties with the back and forth of conversation' 'Frequently talking at length about a favorite subject without noticing that others are not interested or without giving others a chance to respond' 'Displaying facial expressions, movements, and gestures

Having difficulty comprehending or anticipating another person's actions, as well as difficulties adapting to various social settings, difficulties sharing in imaginative play, and difficulties making friends are examples of restrictive or repetitive behaviors.

Having a persistently intense interest in particular topics, such as numbers, details, or facts Showing overly focused interests, such as with moving objects or with parts of objects, Becoming upset by little changes in a routine and having issues with transitions, Being more detective or less detective than other people to sensory input, such as light, sound, clothing, or temperature Being more sensitive or less sensitive than other people to sensory input, such as temperature.

As well, people on the autism spectrum may have a number of strengths, such as:

Being able to learn quickly and retain information for extended periods of time, being adept visual and auditory learners, and excelling in mathematics, science, music, or art are all qualities.

A neurodevelopmental disorder called autism is characterized by:

Autism is a spectrum disorder that affects people of all ethnicities, socioeconomic backgrounds, and ages. It can range from very mild to very severe and cause problems with communication and repetitive behaviors. Autism is four times more common in men than it is in women. Before the age of one or two, some children with autism appear normal, but then suddenly "regress," losing the language or social skills they had previously acquired. The term for this is "regressive" autism.

Initial Signs:

An individual with ASD might:

People with autism may also: Not respond to their name (the child may appear deaf); Not point at objects or things of interest or show interest; Not play "pretend" games; Not make eye contact; Not want to be alone; Have difficulty understanding or showing understanding of other people's feelings or their own; Have no speech or delayed speech; Repeating words or phrases over and again (echolalia); Giving unrelated answers to questions; Getting upset by irrelevant changes; Having obsessive interests; Having irregular reactions.

Excessive anxiety and phobias, as well as unusual phobias Have unusual interests and behaviors Line up toys or other objects Play with toys in the same way every time Like parts of objects (like wheels) Become upset by small changes Have obsessive interests

Unusual eating and sleeping habits Unusual mood or emotional reactions Unusual mood or emotional reactions Lack of fear or more fear than expected Have unusual sleeping habits M-CHAT-RTM General Information The Modified Checklist for Autism in Toddlers, Revised with Follow-Up (M-CHAT-R/F; It is a two-stage parent-report screening tool for Autism Spectrum Disorder (ASD) risk assessment (Robins, Fein, & Barton, 2009). The M-CHAT-R/F is a tool for autism screening that looks for children between the ages of 16 and 30 months who should get a more in-depth evaluation for signs of autism spectrum disorder (ASD) or developmental delay.

All children should undergo broad developmental screenings at ages 9, 18, and 24 months, as well as autism-specific screenings at 18 and 24 months, according to the American Academy of Pediatrics (AAP). At these well-child visits, the M-CHAT-R/F, one of the tools recommended by the AAP, can be administered.

A free developmental assessment can be requested through your state's Department of Health if you and your doctor agree that additional screening is required.

Types of Autism

Autism: When the term "autism" is mentioned, it frequently conjures up images of an individual. These preconceived notions may be accurate for some individuals with Autism; however, not all individuals fall into the category of "classic Autistic."

Autism frequently manifests itself first and foremost during a child's most crucial developmental years, from ages 0 to 6. Parents and other members of the family may become concerned when their children fail to reach certain age-appropriate milestones at these ages.

Because no two cases are the same, the symptoms and signs of autism spectrum disorder will differ from person to person.

There are three distinct types of autism spectrum disorders, which are also referred to as ASD. Find out more about each type of autism and how to identify it in the following paragraphs.

1. Disorder of Autism

Disorder of Autism, also referred to as the "classic case of Autism." When people think of an autistic person, this is typically the scenario that comes to mind. These people may have difficulty communicating verbally and nonverbally, which may cause them to speak slowly, not make facial expressions, or have trouble keeping eye contact while speaking. They might also be hyposensitive to touch, taste, sound, smell, or sight. A person with classic autism may have a negative reaction when either routine or repetition are taken away from them, and it may be difficult for them to go through the motions of everyday life without them. Because they may not be able to empathize with the feelings of other people because they do not experience the same emotions, they may also have difficulty relating to society and other people.

2. **Asperger Syndrome:** Asperger Syndrome is a type of Autism that causes a person to have difficulties in social situations as well as in their behavior or interests. They may have symptoms that are less severe than those of classic autism, but they still face challenges every day. When in social situations, someone with Asperger Syndrome may behave in an inappropriate manner, coming across as awkward or rude. They may appear to be uncaring and self-centered because they feel more at ease talking about themselves than about the person with whom they are interacting. A person with Asperger Syndrome may also have trouble communicating nonverbally, which can make it difficult for them to use the right facial expressions, body language, and gestures.

3. **Pervasive Developmental Disorder**

The term "pervasive developmental disorder-not otherwise specified" (PDD-NOS) refers to people who do not fall under the categories of "autistic disorder" or "asperger syndrome." This person may exhibit high functioning characteristics in addition to mild symptoms of both types of autism. There are three possible categories for these people: high functioning, with symptoms that are similar to those of autism but not quite as severe as autism, and the third group, which includes people who meet all of the criteria for autism but have only mild behavioral symptoms. Since it has only been included in the autism spectrum for the past 15 years, this particular subcategory is relatively new.

Throughout their life, an individual with autism spectrum disorder will face a number of challenges, including those related to social behavior and characteristics, motor functions, and overall behavior patterns. Throughout their life, an individual on the autism spectrum may encounter the following challenges and difficulties.

Activities, interests, and behavior:

Continually performing the same actions, such as rocking back and forth, clapping their hands, or stomping their feet. These movements are frequently performed in a state of relaxation or as a coping strategy.

It may appear out of the ordinary to move in certain ways, like being too rough with a simple hug or being too aggressive when playing with other kids.

It's not uncommon to act or think in a certain way that is obsessive. They might be obsessed with a particular person, a favorite toy, or a particular area of the house. A breakdown, typically accompanied by crying, screams, or tantrums, may occur if this object or person is not present.

It is possible to avoid bringing up other topics of conversation by concentrating on a single subject at all times. People on the Autism spectrum frequently obsess over a particular subject, such as trains or airplanes. They may have a very hard time having a conversation about anything other than the thing they are interested in.

The degree of sensitivity to particular sensory experiences can vary. Some people are extremely sensitive to cold, textures, sounds, and other sensations. while others aren't sensitive enough to them.

Motor skills

There is no one-size-fits-all diagnosis of autism spectrum disorder. Motor skills will vary depending on the severity of the person's autism and any programs or therapy they participate in to avoid these problems. The following are some possible effects on their motor skills:

It's possible for children with autism spectrum disorder to never speak at all or to learn to speak slowly. Although delayed speech after the age of two is one of the first symptoms of Autism Spectrum Disorder, the average age at which a child learns to speak is around two years old.

A person who is able to communicate but also has autism spectrum disorder may frequently repeat a particular phrase and speak at an abnormal volume or tone of voice. They might not know how to talk in the right way, at the right volume, or in the right way.

People with ASD may find it difficult to carry on conversations because they may be frustrated that they are unable to fully express their feelings to those with whom they are speaking. It's possible that they won't be able to comprehend what they're hearing or how to respond to the conversation.

Understanding sarcasm, humor, and literal statements can be challenging for people with ASD, particularly Asperger Syndrome. Contrarily, they might have trouble conveying their sense of humor and come across as rude or rude.

Social Behavior and Characteristics

Similar to how motor skills vary depending on the severity of ASD, social behavior also varies. With the right therapy and professional intervention, social skills can get better over time. Among the social behaviors that may indicate autism spectrum disorder are:

rough play, hitting, scratching, or inappropriate aggression toward peers are examples of aggressive social behavior.

For people with ASD, inappropriate language, actions, or gestures may be common. Lewd language, aggressive or sexual gestures, or actions that are inappropriate for the circumstance they are in are examples of inappropriate behaviors.

A person with ASD can easily misinterpret their feelings, actions, and body language. They might respond in the same way if they take a sentence or action out of context.

Autism spectrum individuals may appear awkward or uncomfortable in social situations. They may react timidly or hostilely to social interactions and likely will not engage in any kind of independent social activity.

It is essential to keep in mind that, although these are typical symptoms of autism spectrum disorder, they are not the only sign of autism. It is essential to understand that a person is not necessarily autistic or on the spectrum just because they possess one of these traits. We encourage you to talk to the person's doctor, family members, and close friends if you think they have autism or are on the spectrum. The only members of society who are legally able to diagnose autism are medical professionals.

We sincerely hope that this information will assist you in distinguishing between the three distinct types of autism. We want to encourage you to treat everyone with the same respect and embrace them regardless of their disability. We believe that each person is just as special and important to us!

Chapter two:
Factors causing and contributing to Autism

Causes of Autism

The question of what causes autism is frequently asked after a diagnosis.

We are aware that autism does not have a single cause. Autism is thought to be the result of a combination of genetic and nongenetic, or environmental, factors.

It would appear that these influences raise a child's risk of developing autism. Nevertheless, it is essential to keep in mind that an increased risk is not the same as a cause. Some gene changes, for instance, that are linked to autism can also be found in people who don't have the condition. In a similar vein, not everyone who is exposed to a risk factor for autism in the environment will develop the disorder. In fact, the majority won't.

Genetic risk

Factors for autism According to research, autism typically runs in families. The risk that a child will develop autism is raised when certain genes are altered. Even if a parent does not have autism, it is possible for one or more of these gene changes to be passed on to a child. Sometimes, these genetic changes happen by themselves in an early embryo or in the sperm and/or egg that form the embryo. Again, the majority of these gene changes do not in and of themselves cause autism. They simply raise the risk of autism.

Environmental risk factors for autism

The research has also shown that certain environmental factors may either raise or lower the risk of autism in people who are genetically predisposed to it. Importantly, none of these risk factors appear to significantly increase or decrease risk:

Pregnancy and birth complications (such as extreme prematurity (before 26 weeks), low birth weight, and multiple pregnancies (twin, triplet, etc.)) are more likely in older parents.

Prenatal vitamins containing folic acid, taken prior to conception, during pregnancy, and afterward have no effect on risk. Vaccinations have no effect on risk. Pregnancies that occur less than a year apart The experience of receiving an autism diagnosis is unique to each family, and for some, it coincides with the timing of their child's vaccinations. In addition, over the course of the past two decades, scientists have conducted extensive research to ascertain whether or not.

Childhood vaccinations are linked to autism.

This study's findings are abundantly clear: Autism is not caused by vaccines. A comprehensive list of this research has been compiled by the American Academy of Pediatrics.

Differences in the biology of the brain

In what ways do these non genetic and genetic factors cause autism? The majority appear to have an impact on important aspects of early brain development. Neurons, or nerve cells, in the brain appear to be affected in some way. Others appear to alter the interconnectedness of entire brain regions. With the intention of developing treatments and supports that can enhance quality of life, research on these differences continues.

Factors contributing to Autism:
(Bringing Light on Autism)
The cause of autism spectrum disorder (ASD) is unknown to medical professionals. There doesn't appear to be a single cause for it. Instead, it's likely that a number of factors combine to make a child more likely to develop these disorders. Some risk factors may be passed down from parents to children. Even before a child is born, the environment that they grow up in may also play a role. The essential information about ASD risk factors can be found here.

 On their porch, a multigenerational Hispanic family displays their family history. Children who have siblings with ASD are more likely to develop autism. The likelihood of having another child with ASD is higher among parents of ASD children. Additionally, relatives of children with autism are more likely to experience minor difficulties in social or communication skills.

Premature Birth

ASD and the nurse Premature Birth ASD can occur before, during, or immediately after birth. Problems during pregnancy may result in premature births. According to research, these issues may be related to ASD. A baby who is born very early before the 26th week of pregnancy may be even more likely to have one of these disorders.

Genes

Genetics may be a factor in why some people get ASD while others don't. When one of the identical twins is affected, 36 to 95% of the time, the other twin will also have ASD, according to research. Additionally, some genetic conditions are associated with autism. A genetic or chromosomal disorder affects about 10% of ASD children. Down syndrome, fragile X syndrome, Tourette's syndrome, and tuberous sclerosis are a few examples. Mutations, or random changes in genes, can also raise the risk of autism.

Using heavy-duty gloves and a high-pressure spray gun, a pest control technician sprays shrubbery Chemicals **Exposure to certain chemicals** before birth may raise an infant's risk of ASD. Pregnant women taking certain medications may be more likely to give birth to children with these conditions. These medicines include thalidomide, which controls mood, valproic acid, which controls seizures, and terbutaline, which prevents preterm labor. Pesticides and chemicals commonly found in plastics (phthalates) may also increase the risk of ASD in unborn children.

Grandmother and child's parents' ages appear to influence a child's risk of ASD. For instance, children born to fathers older than 50 have higher rates of autism. As men get older, there are more genetic mutations in sperm. The increased risk may be explained by this. Also, having a child with ASD is slightly more common in women in their forties. However, there is also an increased risk for babies born to teen moms. The reason why a mother's age affects her child's risk of ASD is unknown to doctors. Couples with ages that are more than 10 years apart are also more likely to have children with autism.

Male ASD affects people of all backgrounds, races, and ethnicities. One of these disorders affects about one in 68 children today, according to health officials. However, boys are more vulnerable than girls. Boys are nearly five times more likely than girls to have ASD.

POLLUTION

Compared to other women, pregnant women who are exposed to high levels of pollution are more likely to have an ASD child. As exposure to pollution rises, so does the risk of autism. When exposure occurs in the final few weeks of pregnancy, this link is strongest. This risk can be increased by a baby's genetic makeup: Children with a particular form of the MET gene and those who were exposed to air pollution before birth are more likely to have autism.

Additional Information There is a widespread misperception that vaccines cause ASD. Thimerosal, a preservative found in vaccines that protect against multiple diseases, has raised some concerns among some individuals. The MMR vaccine, which protects against measles, mumps, and rubella, is of particular concern to them. However, these assertions are unsupported by any scientific evidence. ASD is not caused by vaccines. This superstition has been dispelled by a good number of studies. However, scientists do not yet know what causes ASD. Research in this area is ongoing.

Chapter three:
Therapy and treatment

There are many different kinds of autism therapies that can help people with autism or their families. This kind of therapy also aims to help autistic people become more functionally independent. Level of Evidence (LOE) Level 1 (the highest level assigned based on the methodological quality of their design, validity, and applicability to patient care) does not support the claims made by many therapies marketed toward autistic individuals or their parents. Some facts from a systematic review or meta-analysis of all recognized RCTs (randomized controlled trials) or facts-based clinical practice guidelines based on systematic reviews of RCTs or three or more RCTs of good quality with comparable outcomes are included in Level 1 research. When compared to neurotypical and autistic individuals, autism is a neurotype characterized by differences in sensory and communication abilities. None of these treatments can completely eradicate autism, much less to a high degree of viability. Those who place the elimination of autism ahead of the general well-being of autistic people frequently overlook the fact that autistic children and adults are at risk of burnout and post-traumatic stress disorder (PTSD) caused during childhood and adolescence. Most of the time, treatment is tailored to the person's needs. There are two main types of treatments: medical management and educational interventions. Families of individuals with ASD receive training and assistance as well.

Methodological issues in intervention studies prevent conclusive evaluations of their efficacy. Although there is some evidence that some form of treatment is preferable to no treatment in many psychosocial interventions, systematic reviews have found that the quality of these studies is generally poor, their clinical results are largely inconclusive, and there is little evidence for the relative effectiveness of treatment options. Early intervention in the form of intensive, ongoing special education and behavior therapy can assist children with ASD in developing self-care, social, and employment skills, as well as frequently improve functioning and reduce the severity of symptoms and maladaptive behaviors; Applied behavior analysis (ABA), developmental models, structured teaching, speech and language therapy, social skills therapy, and occupational therapy are some of the methods that are available. When working with autistic children, occupational therapists develop interventions that encourage sharing and cooperation. They also help the autistic child by helping them solve a problem while the occupational therapist imitates the child and waiting for the child to respond. Children benefit from some educational interventions: It is well known that intensive ABA therapy can improve young children's intellectual performance and has been shown to improve global functioning in preschoolers. There is a gap between what a report recommends and what education is provided because neuropsychological reports are frequently poorly communicated to educators. The limited research on adult residential programs' efficacy yields mixed results.

ASD-related issues are treated with a variety of medications. Psychoactive drugs or anticonvulsants are prescribed to more than half of ASD-diagnosed children in the United States. The most common drug classes are stimulants and antidepressants. Aside from antipsychotics, little reliable research has been done on the safety and efficacy of ASD drug treatments for adults and adolescents. There is no known medication that alleviates autism's core symptoms of social and communication impairments, and a person with ASD may respond to medications in unusual ways.

The treatments given to children with ASD were expensive as of 2008; More so are indirect costs. A study conducted in the United States estimated a discounted lifetime cost of $4.66 million (2023 dollars, inflation-adjusted from a 2003 estimate) for a person who was born in the year 2000. This figure includes approximately 10% of the cost of medical care, 30% of the cost of additional education and other care, and 60% of the cost of losing economic productivity. For an autistic person with or without an intellectual disability, a UK study estimated discounted lifetime costs of £1.9 million and £1.23 million, respectively (2023 pounds, inflation-adjusted from 2005/06 estimate). Legal rights to treatment are complicated, depend on where you live and how old you are, and caregivers need to fight for them. Programs funded by the government are frequently insufficient or inappropriate for a particular child, and unreimbursed out-of-pocket medical or therapy costs are linked to the likelihood of family financial difficulties; According to a 2008 U.S. study, families of children with ASD experience an average annual income loss of 14%, and a related study found that ASD is associated with a higher likelihood that issues with child care will significantly impact parental employment. Residential care, job training and placement, sexuality, social skills, and estate planning are important treatment issues after childhood.

Educational intervention

In addition to helping children learn academic subjects and acquire traditional readiness skills, educational interventions aim to improve functional communication and spontaneity, develop cognitive skills like symbolic play, reduce disruptive behavior, and generalize learned skills by applying them to new situations. Several program models have been created, many of which overlap and share many features in practice, such as:

early treatment that doesn't require a definitive diagnosis;
intensive treatment, at least 25 hours per week, year-round;
low teacher-to-student ratio;
involvement in the family, including parental education;
interaction with peers who are neurotypical;
social stories, ABA, and other training that uses pictures;
structure with a routine that is predictable and physical boundaries that are clear to prevent distractions; and ongoing evaluation of a meticulously planned intervention, resulting in any necessary adjustments.

There are a number of options for educational intervention, which are outlined below. They can occur at a center for autism treatment, at a school, or at home; Parents, teachers, speech-language pathologists, and occupational therapists can all use them. A 2007 study found that a special education teacher's weekly home visits augmented a center-based program to improve cognitive development and behavior.

Methodological flaws in intervention studies prevent definitive conclusions regarding efficacy. Although there is some evidence to suggest that some form of treatment is preferable to no treatment in many psychosocial interventions, the methodological quality of these studies' systematic reviews has generally been poor, their clinical results are typically inconclusive, and there is little evidence for the relative effectiveness of various treatment options. The most significant factor in determining how scientific studies' outcomes are interpreted is a concern about outcome measures, such as their inconsistent use. According to a 2009 study conducted in Minnesota, parents adhere to recommendations for behavioral treatment significantly less frequently than they do to medical recommendations, and they adhere more frequently to recommendations for reinforcement than to recommendations for punishment. Early intervention with behavior therapy and intensive, ongoing special education can help children learn self-care, social, and job skills, improve functioning, and often reduce the severity of symptoms and maladaptive behaviors; There is no evidence to support claims that intervention is essential before the age of three.

There have been three major national education policies in the United States that have dealt with special education. The Individuals with Disabilities Education Act of 1997, the Education for All Handicapped Children Act of 1975, and the No Child Left Behind Act of 2001 were examples of these laws. The development of those policies revealed expanded requirements and guidelines for special education; such as requiring additional qualifications for special education teachers, creating a more specialized classroom environment for students with disabilities, ensuring that all students have equal access to opportunities, assisting with postsecondary transitions, and requiring states to fund special education. Special education was significantly impacted by the Individuals with Disabilities Education Act, which mandated that public schools hire highly qualified staff. In 2009, the following were necessary to become a Certified Autism Specialist: a master's degree, two years of professional experience working with people with autism, 14 hours of annual continuing education in autism, and registration with the International Institute of Education

Martha Nussbaum discusses how education is one of the fertile functions that is important for the development of a person and their ability to achieve a multitude of other capabilities within society. She also discusses the perceived disadvantages of autistic people in the United States in the 2010s. Deficits in imitation, observational learning, and receptive and expressive communication are among the many symptoms of autism that hinder a child's ability to receive an appropriate education. As of 2014, autism ranked third lowest among all disabilities in terms of acceptance into postsecondary institutions. Shattuck et al. conducted a 2012 study with funding from the National Institutes of Health. found that, in comparison to 40% of children with a learning disability, only 35% of autistic children enroll in a two- or four-year college within the first two years of high school. This statistic demonstrates that autistic people are at a disadvantage in acquiring many of the skills discussed by Nussbaum and makes education more than just a form of therapy for those with autism because of the growing requirement for a college education to get a job. Shattuck's study from 2012 found that only 55% of children with autism worked for money in the first two years after high school. Additionally, people with autism who come from low-income families are less likely to succeed in postsecondary education.

Schools frequently lacked the resources necessary to create what was then thought to be the ideal classroom environment for students "in need of special education." Educating an autistic child may cost an additional $6,595 to $10,421 in the United States in 2014. The average cost of a public school education for a student in the 2011–2012 academic year was $12,401. In some instances in 2015, the cost of educating an autistic child nearly doubled that of the typical public school student. It is extremely challenging to develop an autism program that is well-suited to the entire population of autistic people as well as those with other disabilities due to the wide range of individuals with autism. In 2014, many school districts in the United States mandated that all schools meet the needs of disabled students, regardless of the number of disabled students enrolled. The special education system is lacking as a result of this and a lack of licensed special education teachers. Some states issued temporary special education licenses to teachers in 2011 as a result of the shortage, with the condition that they obtain permanent licenses within a few years.

Mexico passed a law requiring the inclusion of people with disabilities in education in 1993. Although this law was very important to education in Mexico, its implementation has been difficult due to a lack of resources.

Internationally and through the United Nations Numerous international organizations have also published reports that address issues related to special education. "International Norms and Standards relating to Disability" in 1998 by the United Nations. This report refers to various shows, explanations, statements, and different reports, for example, The Salamanca Statement, the Sundberg Declaration, the Copenhagen Declaration and Programme of Action, and a lot of other documents. The report emphasizes, among other things, that education must be a human right. The quality of education should be the same to that of individuals without disabilities, the report adds. The report also addresses integrated education, supplementary special education classes, teacher education, and equality for vocational education. A report by the Special Rapporteur that focuses on people with disabilities is also published by the United Nations. Result of the research carried out by the Special Rapporteur to the 52nd Session of the Commission for Social Development: was published in 2015 as a report. The publication of the "Note by the Secretary-General on Monitoring the Implementation of the Standard Rules on the Equalization of Opportunities for Persons with Disabilities" occurred. The many countries involved were examined in this report, with an emphasis on Africa, to see how they have implemented disability policy. The author also emphasizes the significance of education for people with disabilities and policies that have the potential to enhance the education system, such as a shift toward a more inclusive approach, in this discussion. In their 2011 "World Report on Disability," the World Health Organization has also published a report on people with disabilities. Within this report, education is discussed. The World Bank, UNICEF, and UNESCO are some of the other organizations that have published reports on the subject.

Environmental enrichment

The way the brain is affected by the stimulation of its information processing provided by its surroundings (including the opportunity to interact socially) is the focus of environmental enrichment. In environments that are richer and more stimulating, brains have more synapses and dendrite arbors that are more complex. This effect occurs mostly during neurodevelopment, but less frequently in adulthood as well. In addition, increased synapse activity results in an increase in the size and number of glial energy-support cells. In order to provide the neurons and glial cells with additional energy, capillary vasculature is also increased. The neurons, glial cells, and capillaries that make up the neuropil expand, making the cortex thicker. Additionally, there may be additional neurons, at least in rodents.

According to studies conducted on nonhuman animals, environments that are more stimulating may aid in the treatment and recovery of a wide range of brain-related disorders, such as Alzheimer's disease and those associated with aging, whereas environments that are devoid of stimulation may hinder cognitive development.

According to human research, deprivation such as in traditional orphanages causes cognitive delay and impairment. Higher levels of education, which are both associated with people engaging in more challenging cognitive activities and are themselves cognitively stimulating, are found to increase resilience (cognitive reserve) to the effects of aging and dementia, according to research.

Massage therapy

A review of massage therapy as a treatment for autism symptoms found that there was little benefit. Music Therapy uses elements of music to allow people to express their feelings and communicate. There were few high-quality studies, and due to the risk of bias found in the analyzed studies, no definitive conclusions regarding the efficacy of massage therapy[98]. According to a review published in 2014 and updated in 2022, music therapy may facilitate social interactions and communication.

Depending on where the patient is on the ASD scale, different methods can be used in music therapy. On the ASD scale, a person who is "high-functioning" would require significantly different treatment than a person who is "low-functioning." The following are examples of these kinds of therapeutic methods:

Performing or recreating music, reproduction of a pre-composed piece of music or song with associated activities Composing music or creating music that caters to some specific needs of that individual using instruments or the voice Listening engaged in specific musical listening base exercises Improvisational music therapy (IMT) is becoming increasingly popular as a therapeutic method being applied to children with autism spectrum disorder (ASD). Using a variety of instruments, song, and movement, the client and therapist create music during the IMT process. Each child or client's unique requirements must be taken into consideration. IMT sessions need to have a certain routine and be predictable in their interactions and surroundings because some children with ASD find their various environments to be chaotic and confusing. All of these things can be provided by music: it can be very predictable, its melodies and sounds are very repetitive, and it can be easily varied with phrasing, rhythm, and dynamics, giving it controlled flexibility. The child may feel more at ease and activities can be incorporated into everyday life when parents or other caregivers are allowed to attend sessions.

Sensory enrichment therapy

The primary goal of any intervention for autistic children is to increase sensitivity across all senses. Most of the time, autistic children don't know how to interpret their senses and the emotions and moods of others. This Sensory Processing Disorder affects a large number of children with autism. After participating in sensory-based therapies for some time, there have been signs of improvement in the children's ability to respond appropriately to stimuli. However, there is currently no solid evidence to suggest that these therapies are beneficial to children with autism. Autism is a very complicated condition that is unique to each child. Because of this, not every form of therapy or therapy activity is equally effective.

These differentiated interventions aim to intervene at the neurological level of the brain in the hope of developing appropriate responses to the various body sensations and environmental stimuli. Music therapies, massage therapies, occupational therapies, and others have all been utilized by scientists. Each situation is unique because the Autistic Spectrum is so wide-ranging and diverse.

A recent systematic review provides support for the emerging evidence that mindfulness-based interventions can improve adults with autism's mental health. This includes evidence that stress, anxiety, ruminating, rage, and aggression can be reduced.

Parent-mediated intervention

Parents of autistic children can get support and advice from parent-mediated interventions. A Cochrane Review conducted in 2013 discovered that although there was strong evidence for a positive pattern of change in parent-child interactions, there was no evidence of gains in the majority of the primary measures of the studies (such as the child's adaptive behavior). The child's language and communication had changed in some ambiguous ways. Although a small number of randomized and controlled studies suggest that parent training can reduce maternal depression, increase maternal understanding of autism and communication styles, and enhance child communicative behavior, no conclusive proof of its efficacy is available due to the design and number of studies.

Children with ASD can often be identified early, before they reach the age of three. A child with ASD's quality of life can be impacted by strategies that focus on early behavior. To best support their child's growth, parents can learn interaction and behavior management techniques. Parent intervention resulted in some improvements, according to a 2013 Cochrane review.

Medical management

In an effort to alleviate common autistic symptoms like seizures, insomnia, irritability, and hyperactivity—which can make it difficult for autistic people to adjust to society or school—drugs, supplements, or diets are frequently used to alter physiology. Medical treatment is supported by a lot of anecdotal evidence; There are a few well-publicized reports of children who are able to return to mainstream education after treatment, with significant improvements in health and well-being. Additionally, many parents who try one or more therapies report some progress. However, the difficulty of verifying reports of improvements, the lack of reporting of treatments' negative outcomes, and the improvements seen in autistic children who grow up without treatment may distort this evidence. Using controlled experiments, only a small number of medical treatments are supported by scientific evidence.

Medication:

A lot of medications are used to treat ASD-related issues. Psychoactive drugs or anticonvulsants are prescribed to more than half of ASD-diagnosed children in the United States. The most common drug classes are antidepressants, stimulants, and antipsychotics. Only antipsychotics have been shown to be effective.

LSD was studied from the 1950s to the 1970s, but it has not been studied in this way since.

A lot of research has been done on atypical antipsychotics, particularly risperidone, which has the most evidence of consistently showing improvements in ASD symptoms like irritability, self-injury, aggression, and tantrums. The Food and Drug Administration (FDA) has approved the use of risperidone to treat autistic children and adolescents with symptomatic irritability. The majority of adverse events in short-term trials (up to six months) were mild to moderate, and monitoring was required for weight gain, drowsiness, and high blood sugar; Long-term safety and efficacy have not been completely established. Risperidone's effect on autism's fundamental social and communication deficits is unknown. A study of autistic children with severe and persistent issues with tantrums, aggression, and self-injury formed part of the FDA's decision; Risperidone should not be used on autistic children who exhibit sporadic explosive behavior and mild aggression.

In the United States, other medications are prescribed without a prescription, meaning that they are not approved for ASD treatment. At the beginning of 2008, massive placebo-controlled studies of olanzapine and aripiprazole were in progress. Aripiprazole has been linked to side effects like weight gain and sedation, but it may be effective for the short term in treating autism.

Dopamine blockers and selective serotonin reuptake inhibitors (SSRIs) can reduce some of the atypical behaviors that come with ASD. A 2009 multisite randomized controlled study found no benefit and some adverse effects from the SSRI citalopram in children, despite the fact that SSRIs reduce levels of repetitive behavior in autistic adults. This raises questions about whether SSRIs are effective for treating repetitive behavior in autistic children. The prescription of SSRI antidepressants for the treatment of autistic spectrum disorders in children lacked any evidence, so it could not be recommended, according to a subsequent study of related medical reviews.

The psychostimulant methylphenidate may be effective against ASD hyperactivity and possibly impulsivity, according to reviews of the evidence, despite the fact that the findings were limited by low-quality evidence. "Has a negative impact on the core symptoms of ASD, or that it improves social interaction, stereotypical behaviors, or overall ASD," according to the study, "has no evidence." Only risperidone and methylphenidate have demonstrated results that have been replicated out of the numerous medications that have been studied for the treatment of aggressive and self-injurious behavior in children and adolescents with autism.

In 1998, a study on the hormone secretin found that it helped with symptoms, which sparked a lot of interest. However, subsequent controlled studies have found no benefit. In rodents, an experimental drug called STX107 stopped the overproduction of metabotropic glutamate receptor 5. It has been hypothesized that this may help in about 5% of cases of autism, but this hypothesis has not been tested in humans.

Oxytocin may be a treatment option for repetitive and affiliative behaviors and may play a role in autism; Oxytocin improves emotion interpretation and reduced repetitive behavior, according to two related studies on adults; however, these preliminary findings may not necessarily apply to children. Oxytocin, according to recent research, may make the brain's auditory system quieter, making it easier to perceive social cues and react appropriately in social situations. However, not all of the detected cues are positive: While increasing awareness of an aggressor may cause distress, increasing awareness of a trusted adult may be beneficial. Oxytocin's use as a treatment for autism spectrum disorder should be closely monitored due to the possibility that its effects are context-dependent.

Aside from antipsychotics, little reliable research has been done on the safety and efficacy of ASD drug treatments for adults and adolescents. The few randomized controlled trials that have been conducted indicate that the opioid antagonist naltrexone hydrochloride is ineffective and that risperidone, the SSRI fluvoxamine, and the common antipsychotic haloperidol may be more effective than the tricyclic antidepressant clomipramine in reducing some behaviors. Memantine has been shown to significantly improve social behavior and language function in children with autism in small studies. Memantine's effects on adults with autism spectrum disorders are the subject of ongoing research. It is possible for a person with ASD to react abnormally to medications, and these medications may also cause undesirable side effects.

Prosthetics In contrast to standard neuromotor prosthesis, neurocognitive prostheses would physically reconstitute cognitive processes like language and executive function by sensing or modifying neural function. Although implantable neurocognitive brain-computer interfaces have been proposed as a means of assisting in the treatment of conditions such as autism, there are currently no neurocognitive prostheses available.

It has been suggested that autistic people can improve their social communication skills by using affective computing devices, typically equipped with image or voice recognition capabilities. The development of these devices is still ongoing. Additionally, the use of robots as educational tools for children with autism has been proposed.

Transcranial magnetic stimulation, a treatment for depression that is somewhat well-established, has been proposed and utilized as a treatment for autism. There was insufficient evidence to support its widespread use for autism spectrum disorders, according to a 2013 review. A review conducted in 2015 uncovered preliminary but insufficient evidence to support its use outside of clinical studies. TMS can positively influence gamma brainwave oscillations and help improve performance accuracy, according to new research.

Medicine alternative

In the 1990s and early 2000s, a number of alternative treatments and approaches, such as elimination diets and chelation therapy, were popular, but few of them were supported by scientific studies. In quality-of-life contexts, treatment approaches lacked empirical support, and many programs focused on success metrics that lacked predictive validity and real-world relevance. Program marketing, training availability, and parent requests appeared to be more important to service providers than scientific evidence. Back then, it was assumed that conservative treatments like diet changes were "expected to be harmless aside from their brother and cost" even if they didn't help. However, this didn't take into account the negative impact on the mental health of the children in question, who are now adults who are speaking out against such practices.

Acupuncture

Acupuncture was investigated, but it was not found to be "helpful in treating autism."

Hyperbaric oxygen

A boy with ASD and his father in a chamber filled with hyperbaric oxygen. Photo submitted in 2005) In 2007, additional studies were required for practitioners and families to make decisions regarding HBOT treatments that were more conclusive and valid. Although this study has not been independently verified, a small 2009 double-blind study of autistic children found that 40 hourly treatments of 24% oxygen at 1.3 atmospheres significantly improved the children's behavior immediately following treatment sessions. Since then, a number of relatively large controlled studies have been conducted to investigate HBOT. For instance, in 2010, treatments utilizing 24% oxygen at 1.3 atmospheres yielded less encouraging results. In a 2010 double-blind study, children with autism were given either HBOT or a placebo. The treatment was evaluated using both standardized psychological assessments and direct observational measures of behavioral symptoms. On any outcome measure, there were no differences found between the HBOT group and the placebo group. Using multiple baselines from 16 participants, a second single-subject study conducted in 2011 also examined the effects of 40 HBOT treatments containing 24% oxygen at 1.3 atmospheres on directly observed behaviors. Again, there were no consistent results across any group, and there were also no significant improvements in any one participant. These studies, taken together, suggest that HBOT at 24% oxygen and 1.3 atmosphere pressure does not significantly improve autistic disorder behavioral symptoms. Nevertheless, reports in the media and related blogs indicated that HBOT was utilized for numerous autism-related cases in the 2010s.

HBOT appears to be riskier and, consequently, frequently less favorable when taking into account the inconsistent findings, as well as the financial and time commitments required to participate in this treatment. As of May 2011, HBOT could cost up to $150 per hour for people who use it as part of their integrated treatment programs for 40 to 120 hours. The HBOT chambers can also be purchased (for $8,495–27,995) or rented ($1,395 per month) by some families.

Hyperbaric oxygen therapy provides a higher concentration of oxygen that is delivered in a chamber or tube containing atmospheric pressure that is higher than sea level, as of 2017. There is no evidence in case series or randomized controlled trials that HBOT is beneficial for ASD children. This treatment was only found to be effective in one randomized controlled trial, and no other studies have replicated those findings.

Chiropractic is a form of alternative medicine in which spinal manipulation is the main treatment and the main hypothesis is that mechanical disorders of the spine affect overall health through the nervous system. Because traditional chiropractic philosophy compares vaccines to poison, a significant portion of the profession opposes vaccination. The majority of chiropractic writings on vaccination focus on its negative aspects, asserting that it is risky, ineffective, and unnecessary. In some cases, they also suggest that vaccination causes autism or that chiropractors should be the primary source of treatment for neurodevelopmental disorders like autism. For medical conditions other than back pain, chiropractic care has not been shown to be effective, and there is insufficient scientific evidence to draw conclusions regarding chiropractic care for autism.

Craniosacral therapy is a form of alternative medicine based on the idea that gentle pressure applied to external areas can improve the flow and balance of the supply of cerebrospinal fluid to the brain, alleviating symptoms of a variety of conditions, and that restrictions at cranial sutures of the skull affect rhythmic impulses conveyed via cerebrospinal fluid. There is little scientific evidence to support the therapy, there is no scientific support for major components of the underlying model, and research methods that could definitively evaluate the therapy's effectiveness have not been utilized. There are no published studies on this therapy's use for autism.

Chelation therapy

Some parents have turned to alternative medicine practitioners who offer detoxification treatments through chelation therapy because it is possible that heavy metal poisoning can cause autism symptoms, particularly in small groups of people who are unable to eliminate toxins effectively. However, there has been little rigorous evidence to support this practice. Strong epidemiological evidence disproves the existence of links between the onset of autistic symptoms and environmental triggers, particularly vaccines containing thimerosal. In 2002, it was hypothesized that thiamine tetrahydrofurfuryl disulfide (TTFD) could be used as a chelating agent in children with autism. A pilot study administered TTFD directly to ten children on the autism spectrum in 2002, and it appeared to have a positive clinical effect. A 2006 review of thiamine by the same author did not mention the possibility of thiamine having an impact on autism, and this study has not been replicated. The use of thiamine (vitamin B1) as a treatment for autism is not supported by sufficient evidence. The problem with questionable invasive treatments is much more serious: For instance, an unsuccessful chelation therapy in 2005 resulted in the death of an autistic 5-year-old boy.

The claim that the mercury in the vaccine preservative thimerosal causes autism or its symptoms is not supported by any scientific data, and chelation therapy as a treatment for autism is not supported by any scientific data either.

Hypotheses about diets and supplements

In the 1990s At the beginning of that decade, it was hypothesized that opioid peptides like casomorphin, which are metabolic products of gluten and casein, could either cause or exacerbate autism. Diets that eliminate foods that contain gluten, casein, or both are widely promoted based on this hypothesis. There are numerous testimonials describing benefits for autism-related symptoms, particularly social engagement and verbal skills. Due to the significant flaws in the studies that supported those claims, the data were insufficient to guide treatment recommendations. In a small 1993 study, stereotyped behavior was reduced by vitamin C. As of 2005, the study had not been replicated, and vitamin C was not widely used as an autism treatment. Kidney stones and gastrointestinal problems like diarrhea may occur at high doses.

Hypotheses and research from 2000 to 2014 In the early 2000s, many parents tried to "treat autism" or "alleviate its symptoms" by giving their children dietary supplements. There were many supplements offered, but only a few are supported by scientific evidence.

In 2005, it was believed: Even though some children with autism also have gastrointestinal (GI) symptoms, there isn't enough rigorous data that has been published to support the idea that autistic kids have more or different GI symptoms than usual; There is a lack of clarity regarding the connection between GI issues and ASD and the results of various studies. Atypical eating behavior was once considered a diagnostic indicator because it was thought to occur in approximately three-quarters of ASD children. Although eating rituals and food refusal are also problems, selective eating is the most common one; At the time, studies did not appear to show that it caused malnutrition.

Salicylates, food dyes, yeast, and simple sugars were the targets of additional elimination diets that were suggested. The effectiveness of such diets in "treating autism" in children has not been established by scientific evidence. If proper nutrition is not ensured, an elimination diet may result in nutritional deficiencies that harm overall health.

According to studies from 2006, children with chronic illnesses use complementary and alternative medical (CAM) therapy more frequently than children in the general population. Helen H. L. Wong and Ronald G. Smith conducted a study to compare the patterns of CAM therapy use among children with autism spectrum disorders (n = 50) and a control group of children without ASD (n = 50). 52% of parents in the ASD group reported using or having used at least one complementary and alternative medicine (CAM) therapy for their child, compared to 28% in the control group (P = 0.024). Parents believed that 75% of the therapies used were beneficial, and biologically based therapies like special diets or supplements made up 75% of the therapies used in the ASD group.

For instance, a 2008 study found that autistic boys on a casein-free diet had significantly thinner bones than usual, likely as a result of calcium and vitamin D deficiencies caused by the diet. A 2009 review noted the potential risk of fatal hypermagnesemia and found some low-quality evidence to support the use of vitamin B6 and magnesium in high doses. However, the evidence was ambiguous. Due to the little number of research, the methodological quality of studies, and little sample sizes, no recommendation can be advanced pertaining to the use of B6-Mg as a treatment for autism, according to a 2005 Cochrane Research of the evidence for the usage of B6 and magnesium.

By reducing yeast overgrowth in the colon, probiotics with potentially beneficial bacteria were hypothesized to "relieve some symptoms of autism." Endoscopy has not confirmed the hypothesized yeast overgrowth, the mechanism linking yeast overgrowth to autism is only speculative, and no clinical trials had been published in the peer-reviewed literature as of 2005.

Dimethylglycine (DMG), a common supplement, was thought to "reduce autistic behaviors" and improve speech. There was no statistically significant effect on "autistic behaviors" in two placebo-controlled, double-blind studies, and no peer-reviewed studies have addressed treatment with the related compound trimethylglycine.

Melatonin is occasionally used to treat insomnia. The majority of adverse effects, such as drowsiness, headache, dizziness, and nausea, were reported to be mild. However, susceptible children reported an increase in seizure frequency. Melatonin was found to be effective in treating autistic children's insomnia in a number of small RCTs, but larger studies are needed. "The administration of exogenous melatonin for abnormal sleep parameters in ASD is evidence-based," a 2013 literature review stated, citing 20 studies that reported improvements in sleep parameters as a result of melatonin supplementation.

In spite of the fact that omega-3 fatty acids, also known as polyunsaturated fatty acids (PUFAs), were "a popular treatment for children with ASD" in the 2000s and 2010s, there is very little high-quality scientific evidence to support their efficacy. BDTH2, carnosine, cholesterol, cyproheptadine, D-cycloserine, folic acid, glutathione, metallothionein promoters, other PUFA like omega-6 fatty acids, tryptophan, tyrosine, thiamine (see Chelation therapy), vitamin B12, and zinc were all hypothesized to relieve autism symptoms. These lack dependable scientific facts of autism treatment efficacy or safety.

According to the Mayo Clinic website in 2019, "Yes, children with autism spectrum disorder (ASD) tend to have more medical issues, including gastrointestinal (GI) symptoms such as abdominal pain, constipation, and diarrhea, compared to their peers," it is now known that "children with ASD are at risk of having alimentary tract disorders – primarily, they are at a greater risk of general gastrointestinal (GI) concerns, constipation, diarrhea, and abdominal pain." At this time, there is no "diet for autism," just advice to avoid eating things that the person seems to reject, like: gluten, if the individual has celiac disease. "There is no clinical evidence for applying specific (e.g., gluten-free or probiotic) diets" to the issue of autism as of the year 2021.

Electroconvulsive therapy
Studies conducted in 2009 revealed that 12–17% of autistic adolescents and young adults meet the diagnostic criteria for catatonia, or loss of or excessive motor activity. Catatonia and related conditions in people with autism have been treated with electroconvulsive therapy (ECT), but no controlled trials of ECT in autism had been conducted as of 2009, and its use faces significant ethical and legal challenges.

Stem cell therapy from 2007 to 2012 Mesenchymal stem cells and cord blood CD34+ cells were proposed as a treatment for autism in 2007. As of 2012, it was believed that these cells might be a potential treatment in the future. Mesenchymal stem cells have the greatest potential as a treatment for autism because deregulation of the immune system has been linked to the condition. People with autism have an imbalance in NK cells as well as CD3+, CD4+, and CD8+ T cells, indicating changes in the innate immune system as well as the adaptive immune system. Additionally, PBMCs, or mononuclear cells found in the peripheral blood, overproduce IL-1. It was hypothesized that immune suppressive activity mediated by MSCs could correct this immune imbalance.

Other

 Pseudoscience: A few naturopathic doctors say that CEASE therapy, which combines homeopathy, supplements, and "vaccine detoxing," can help people with autism, but there isn't much solid evidence to support this claim.

Children were tightly wrapped in wet, refrigerated sheets for up to an hour during packing, leaving only their heads free. The treatment could continue for years and was repeated several times per week. It was meant to be a treatment for autistic kids who hurt themselves or couldn't talk, mostly. Similar envelopment methods had been used for centuries, such as in the 19th century in Germany to calm violent patients; Based on psychoanalytic theories like the theory of the refrigerator mother, it was revived in France in the 1960s. Packing was used in hundreds of French clinics as of 2007. In 2007, there was no scientific evidence that packing was effective, and there was some concern about the possibility of adverse health effects. As of 2019: " In April 2016, the French Secretary of State made the announcement to the Ministry of Health that "the main French associations of parents with autistic children succeeded in obtaining the prohibition of packing."

Antidotes to autistic burnouts:

The majority of people can think of a time in their lives when they would identify as burnout. This usually means that someone has too much energy for their job or has taken on too many activities in general.

However, the term has taken on a new meaning within the autism community that is exclusive to autistic people. It was described as "a syndrome conceptualized as resulting from chronic life stress and a mismatch of expectations and abilities without adequate support" in a 2020 AASPIRE research study. It is characterized by pervasive, long-term (typically more than three months) exhaustion, function loss, and decreased stimulus tolerance. In contrast to depression, it goes beyond fatigue. Instead, for autistic people, it is a series of experiences that accumulate over time because they are no longer able to handle the responsibilities or expectations in their lives. The person with autism experiences burnout when they lose the skills and abilities they would normally have.

Autistic burnout appears to be exacerbated by striving for social acceptance and neurotypical behavior. Changing one's behavior and impulses to appear more "normal" takes a lot of brain, brain, and emotional energy. Try to picture a pie chart that shows how well you think. When a person alters their social presentation through ongoing self-awareness and self-monitoring, it reduces the cognitive capacity they have available for other tasks. It's important to remember that nobody chooses to burn out. It's a sign of a neurological state that doesn't go away. The individual may notice that they are becoming less capable than usual or that they are having more meltdowns or shutdowns, both of which can indicate that they are beginning to feel burnout. Sometimes, burnout has such a gradual effect on people that they don't realize they're struggling until they're completely incapacitated or until someone else tells them they're not doing so well.

Typically, autistic burnout is characterized by an increase in sensory sensitivity and cognitive difficulty in making decisions and effectively managing tasks, organizing activities, and remembering things. Speaking ability is also negatively impacted for many autistic people. Suicidal thoughts and impulses may also rise in autistic burnout.

If you or someone you care about is experiencing burnout, even though not all episodes of burnout can be avoided, it is essential to have a strategy you can put into action in advance to lessen the likelihood of experiencing burnout. Reduce the intensity and length of the episode when possible at times. Fortunately, there are a number of ways to combat burnout or prevent it if it occurs. The following recommendations are not "one-size-fits-all." Try what makes sense for your situation or that of a loved one.

More is less: Recognize the warning signs if you suspect you are approaching burnout. Try to include more downtime in your schedule to get some relief. While there may be demands from your job, school, or family that you cannot compromise on, anything you can do to give yourself more time for recreation and rest is a positive step toward avoiding burnout. If you can, add more time to sleeping. The majority of people with autism have trouble getting deep sleep, so they may need more time in bed to get the same amount of sleep as a neurotypical person. Your nervous system can benefit from some respite by taking even the tiniest amounts of time throughout the day to allow your eyes to relax and focus on something else for a while.

Encourage your autistic loved one to make time for themselves a priority and find out what they need from you to make life easier for them.

Follow your passions: Autistic people can get a lot of energy from their "special" or "intense" interests, which can also help with burnout prevention or recovery. Make time to sort Magic cards, read a book about art history, or do something creative with your hands. This kind of regenerative activity can support your ability to complete less preferred activities. Additionally, simply perusing your collection of materials related to an intense interest can boost your mood. Even if you don't have the time or space to really pull your belongings out and interact with them, organizing, tidying, and handling them can make you feel better.

By encouraging autistic loved ones to pursue their unique interests, friends, partners, and family can assist. They can also demonstrate their support by interacting with an autistic friend or family member, asking about their interests, participating in those interests with them, or proving their validity in other ways.

Always Learning: Are you experiencing a lack of intense interest right now? Burnout may be a sign if you have lost focus or veered away from your passions and activities. Going to a large bookstore or library and starting to browse is one way to regain your enthusiasm and enthusiasm for life. It's okay to write down book titles at a store and see if you can borrow them from your library or ask for an interlibrary loan if you have a limited budget. If reading books isn't your thing, look for free apps to learn more.

Explore on your own and see what piques your interest. You might get caught up in a topic you didn't expect. You might decide that manga, sailboats, chess, or the history of Latin American weaving interest you. You might also be captivated by other aspects of life that you are unaware of. It's possible that recently published material on a subject you used to be interested in will pique your interest once more.

If you don't like going to libraries or bookstores, there are other options like going to your favorite museums or parks if you like being outside and seeing what draws you there.

If you are unable to leave the house or do not have access to these resources, online research may pique your interest, but it is not as vivid as planning a field trip to the real world.

For those hoping to offer help, you can help by setting aside a few minutes and transportation (if necessary) accessible to your medically introverted cherished one to seek after their interest.

Possibility of Repetition: Stimming is one way that people with autism are different from people who are neurotypical. Everyone stims periodically, like tapping their pen or spinning their hair, however medically introverted individuals have a neurological need to stimulate to deliver energy and self-mitigate. Try to incorporate it into your day in a creative way if you don't want others to see you smoking. Wear fabrics that you can feel and that have pleasant textures. Make sure you keep the pens you really like at your workstation. As you move your fingers across the palms of your hands, quietly wiggle them and count or make patterns.

Accepting the value of stimming and providing an environment where autistic loved ones can freely stim without fear of repercussions can be helpful.

The World of Senses: There are more kinds of sensing than the five that we talk about. The proprioceptive system, for instance, is the knowledge of our body's location in space and in relation to our surroundings. The interoceptive system gives us awareness of our bodies and what they are doing, like feeling hungry or thirsty, needing to get rid of waste, and experiencing emotions. Being autistic can affect any of these functions. Many autistic people struggle with their senses. In fact, for children's sensory processing issues, occupational therapists frequently recommend a "sensory diet," which consists of physical activities and sensory-specific accommodations; Adults who are open to trying new things can use this idea to create their own sensory diet.

You can better deal with burnout or manage it when it starts to creep in by engaging in these activities, which can help you diversify your sensory input. You don't have to live with burnout, so keep trying because different things can help at different times.

and assistance If you have just learned that your child may or may not have autism spectrum disorder, you probably have a lot of questions and anxiety about what to do next. A diagnosis of ASD can be particularly something to be afraid of because no parent is ever prepared to get to know that their kid is not happy and in good health. You might be perplexed by complicated treatment recommendations or not sure of the ways that are more effective to assist your child. Alternatively, you might have been told that ASD is a lifelong, incurable situation, causing you to be worried that there's nothing you can do that will have any effect.

Although ASD is not something that a person simply "grows out of," there are a number of treatments that can assist children in acquiring new skills and overcoming a wide range of developmental obstacles. Assistance for your child's special needs, including in-home behavioral therapy, school-based programs, and free government services, are all available.

Taking care of oneself is just as important as taking care of an autistic child. You can be the best parent you can be to your child in need if you are emotionally strong. Having an autistic child can be made easier with these parenting tips.

As a parent of an individual kid with ASD or related developmental slowness, the better thing you can do is to start treatment the very moment it is diagnosed. Don't wait for a diagnosis. As soon as you think something is wrong, get help. Do not wait to see if your child will catch up in the future or outgrow the issue. Waiting for a formal diagnosis is pointless. Children with autism spectrum disorder have a better chance of completing treatment if they seek help as soon as possible. The best way to speed up your child's development and reduce their autism symptoms over time is through early intervention.

Learning more about autism if your child has it.
ItYou will be better able to make informed decisions for your child if you know more about autism spectrum disorder. Participate in all treatment decisions, educate yourself about the options for treatment, and ask questions.

Learn all you can about your child. Find out what makes your child behave in a challenging or disruptive way and what makes them respond positively. What causes your child anxiety or apprehension? Calming? Uncomfortable? Enjoyable? You'll be better able to solve problems and avoid or alter situations that cause difficulties if you know what affects your child.

Acknowledge your youngster, characteristics what not. Acceptance is more important than focusing on how your autistic child differs from other children or what he or she "misses." Stop comparing your child to others and take pleasure in your child's unique quirks and small accomplishments. Your child will benefit most from experiencing unconditional love and acceptance.

Never give up. The course of autism spectrum disorder cannot be predicted. Don't just go into conclusions yet about what your child's life may be like. People with autism, like everyone else, have a lifetime to grow and develop their abilities.

Tip 1: for helping your autistic child thrive: Ensure your child's safety and structure by learning as much as you can about autism and participating in treatment. Additionally, the following suggestions will make your child with ASD's daily home life easier:

Keep it up. It is difficult for children with ASD to transfer what they have learned in one setting—like the therapist's office or school—to other settings—like the home. For instance, while your child may use sign language at school to communicate, you may never consider it. The most effective way to reinforce learning is to establish consistency in your child's environment. Continue your child's therapist's methods at home by learning about them. If you want to encourage your child to transfer what he or she has learned from one environment to another, look into the possibility of having therapy take place in more than one location. Be consistent in how you interact with your child and respond to challenging behaviors as well.

Follow a schedule. Children with autism typically perform better when they have a strict routine or schedule. This all comes back to the need and desire for consistency. Establish a routine for your child that includes established times for meals, therapy, school, and bedtime.

Always try keeping this prescribed routine as easy and as possible as you can. Your child should be prepared for any unavoidable schedule adjustments in advance.

Reward good conduct. When it comes to children with ASD, positive reinforcement can go a long way, so try to "catch them doing something good." Be very specific about the behavior for which you are praising them and give them praise when they behave appropriately or learn a new skill. Give them a sticker or let them play with a favorite toy as additional ways to reward them for good behavior.

Make a safe area in your home. In your home, create a private area where your child can unwind, feel safe, and secure. This will require organizing and establishing clear boundaries for your child. Visual cues like using colored tape to mark off-limits areas or using pictures to label things in the house can be helpful. If your child is prone to tantrums or other self-injurious behaviors, you may also need to make the house safer.

Tip 2: Connecting with an autistic child can be difficult, but you don't have to talk or even touch in order to connect and communicate. You communicate with your child through the way you look at them, the tone of your voice, your body language, and perhaps even the way you touch them. Even if your child never speaks, he or she is still expressing himself or herself to you. It's just about the mindset of language acquisition.

Find nonverbal clues. You can learn to recognize autistic children's nonverbal communication cues if you are observant and aware. When they are tired, hungry, or in need of something, pay close attention to the sounds they make, their facial expressions, and the gestures they make.

Determine the reason for the tantrum. It is normal to be upset when you are misunderstood or ignored, and children with ASD are no different. When children with ASD act out, it's usually because you don't notice what they're saying. Their method of expressing their dissatisfaction and gaining your attention is to throw a tantrum.

[Read: Problems with Autism's Behaviour] Schedule time for fun. A child with ASD continues to be a child. There must be more to life than therapy for autistic children and their parents. When your child is most alert and awake, schedule playtime. Think about the things that bring your child out of her or his shell and help you come up with ways to have fun together. If these activities do not appear to be educational or therapeutic, it is likely that your child will enjoy them the most. Both your enjoyment of your child's company and your child's enjoyment of unstructured time with you have significant benefits. Every child needs to play as part of their education, and it shouldn't feel like work.

Pay close attention to your child's sensitivities to the senses. Hypersensitivity to light, sound, touch, taste, and smell is common in ASD children. Sensory stimuli can be "under-sensitive" in some children with autism. Find out what sights, sounds, smells, movements, and tactile sensations cause your child to engage in "bad" or disruptive behaviors and what makes them respond positively. What causes your child anxiety? Calming? Uncomfortable? Enjoyable? You'll be better able to solve problems, avoid situations that cause problems, and create positive experiences if you know what influences your child.

Tip 3: Create a customized treatment plan for your child with autism Because there are so many different options, it can be hard to decide which one is best for your child. You might get recommendations from your parents, teachers, and doctors that are not the same or even at odds with each other, which will make things even more complicated.

Keep in mind that there is no one treatment that works for everyone when creating a treatment plan for your child. Each person on the autism spectrum has their own set of abilities and limitations.

The treatment you give your child needs to be specific to them. It is up to you to ensure that your child's needs are met because you know your child best. By asking yourself the following questions, you can accomplish that:

What are my child's advantages and disadvantages?

Which behaviors are presenting the greatest challenges? What essential abilities does my child lack?

My child learns best by doing, watching, or listening.

What activities does my child enjoy, and how can they be utilized in treatment and to enhance learning?

Last but not least, keep in mind that your involvement is essential to success regardless of the treatment plan selected. By working closely with the treatment team and completing the therapy at home, you can help your child get the most out of treatment. This is the reason your health is very important!

A successful treatment plan will:
Take advantage of your child's hobbies.
Provide a regular schedule.
Organize tasks into manageable steps.
Participate actively in highly structured activities with your child.
Reward behavior on a regular basis.
Participate the parents.
Treatment options for autism include behavior therapy, speech-language therapy, physical therapy, occupational therapy, and nutritional therapy, among other options and approaches.

While you don't need to restrict your kid to only each treatment in turn, it's far-fetched that you'll have the option to address everything simultaneously. Instead, focus first on your child's most severe symptoms and immediate requirements.

The assistance in caring for an autistic child can take a lot of time and effort. You might have days when you feel a lot of pressure, stress, or discouragement. Raising a child with special needs is even more difficult than normal. Being a parent is never easy. You must take care of yourself in order to be the best parent you can be.

Do not attempt to perform all tasks independently. There's no need to! Families of children with ASD can get help, support, advocacy, and advice from a variety of sources:

Support groups for ASD: Getting involved in a support group for ASD is a great way to meet other families going through the same struggles as you do. Information and advice can be shared, and parents can rely on one another for emotional support. The isolation that many parents experience after receiving a child's diagnosis can be greatly reduced by simply being around others who are going through the same thing and talking about their experiences.

Care for the sick: Every parent needs a break from time to time. This is especially true for parents dealing with the additional stress of ASD. In respite care, you get a break for a few hours, days, or even weeks while another caregiver takes over temporarily.

Individual, marital, or family counseling: If you're feeling overwhelmed by stress, anxiety, or depression, you might want to see your own therapist. In therapy, you can talk openly about all of your emotions—good, bad, and ugly—in a safe environment. Marriage or family therapy can also assist you in resolving issues that arise in your spousal relationship or with other family members as a result of the difficulties of raising an autistic child.

Services for early intervention (from birth to two years old) The Early Intervention program provides assistance to infants and toddlers from birth to two years old. Your child must first undergo a free evaluation to be eligible. You will collaborate with early intervention treatment providers to create an Individualized Family Service Plan (IFSP) if the assessment reveals a developmental issue. An IFSP specifies the services your child will receive and the requirements they have.

For chemical imbalance, an IFSP would incorporate an assortment of conduct, physical, discourse, and play treatments. It would concentrate on getting autistic children ready for going to school. Early intervention services are typically provided at a child care facility or in the home.

Ask your pediatrician for a referral or use the resources listed in the "Get more help" section at the end of the article to find your child's local early intervention services.

Services in special education for children over the age of three School-based programs provide assistance to children over the age of three. Special education services, like those for early intervention, are tailored to your child's specific requirements. Autistic children are frequently placed in small groups with other children who have developmental delays so that they can receive more individual attention and specialized instruction. However, they may also spend at least some of the school day in a regular classroom, depending on their abilities. The objective is to place children in a "least restrictive environment" where they can still learn.

Your child will first need to be evaluated by the local school system before you can pursue special education services. An Individualized Education Plan (IEP) will be created on the basis of this assessment. Your child's academic objectives for the school year are outlined in an IEP. In addition, it explains the specialized assistance or support your child will receive from the school to achieve those objectives.

Know your rights as a parent of a child with autism spectrum disorder (ASD):

Request an IEP meeting at any time if you feel your child's needs are not being met Free or low-cost legal representation if you can't come to an agreement with the school Caring for a child with autism when you are autistic Research indicates that there is a genetic component to autism. Disagreeing with the recommendations made by the school authority. Seek an outside evaluation for your child. However, many parents only learn that their children are autistic after conducting research and obtaining a formal diagnosis for themselves. When it comes to raising children who are also neurodivergent, being autistic may present unique challenges. Some helpful hints are as follows:

Try not to conceal your personality. Allow your child to discover who you really are. Don't feel pressured to hide your oddities in front of your child if they include repetitive behaviors or unusual body movements. By being yourself, you give your autistic child a chance to connect with you and encourage them to be themselves around you. You can also discuss with your child how neurotypical people might react to your actions and how to deal with negative responses. Try to provide advice that would have been helpful to you when you were younger.

Take care of yourself, always. If you struggle with sensory needs or require a highly structured lifestyle, caring for a child can be difficult. A crying child, for instance, could be a constant source of stress and discomfort for you if you are sensitive to sounds. When your child throws tantrums suddenly, it can be hard to stick to a regular schedule, which only adds to your frustration. It is essential for you to develop coping strategies that assist in reducing your stress in situations like these in order to safeguard your own sense of well-being.

Look to other people for help if some tasks seem too hard. For instance, if it's hard for you to communicate with doctors and teachers, a parenting mentor or other parents of children with autism might be able to help you find solutions.

Make use of your advantages. You are not alone in having particular strengths. Think about how your abilities and skills can help you create a loving home for your child. Do you have a talent for design or visual thinking? Make your child educational posters. Is it safe to say that you are ready to concentrate for extensive stretches of time? Use that focus to learn more about parenting techniques and coping mechanisms. Do you have problem-solving skills? To overcome problems around the house, you can use your imagination and creative thinking outside the box.

Both you and your child require your patience. Accept that you and your partner have plenty of time to grow and learn. It's possible that you'll suffer setbacks. It's possible that you lose your temper and are embarrassed by your response. Or perhaps your child struggles to blend in with their classmates when they start school. Even if you have to try multiple times, make the decision to learn from your mistakes and find solutions. Remember to give credit where credit is due whenever one of you actually makes progress. Give your child praise and acknowledge your own accomplishments.

Chapter four:
Anxiety in autistic kids and adults

What is anxiety?

Anxiety is defined by the NHS as "a feeling of unease that can be mild or severe, such as worry or fear." When it persists for an extended period of time and has a significant impact on a person's life, it becomes a clinical condition.

How can I tell if I'm worried?

Being anxious affects everyone at some particular point in their lives. A change in your daily routine, taking an exam, or going through a job interview may make you feel worried and anxious.

These are signs that you might be anxious:

feeling restless or anxious, a stomach churn, a rapid, thumping, or irregular heartbeat, rapid breathing, sweating, or hot flushes, nausea (feeling sick), difficulty sleeping, or panic attacks.

You may have Generalized Anxiety Disorder (GAD) if your anxiety is persistent, difficult to control, and affecting your daily life. The NHS website has more information about GAD and anxiety.

Why might people with autism feel anxious?

Many people with autism have high levels of anxiety, despite the fact that it is not one of the diagnostic criteria for the disorder. Although the findings of the various studies vary, there is general agreement that around 40 to 50 percent of autistic people may receive a clinical diagnosis of anxiety.

For autistic people, stressful social situations and sensory environments can make them feel even more anxious.

One more huge reason for uneasiness is a feeling of being misjudged as well as not acknowledged by non-mentally unbalanced individuals. Autistic people may disguise or disguise themselves in order to "fit in" and not be noticed as different. This can make them feel more anxious and hurt their mental health.

Anxiety can also be caused by the following other factors:
difficulty recognizing, comprehending, and controlling one's emotions (also referred to as alexithymia) following a change in routine, particularly an unexpected one.
alexithymia).
59% of autistic people polled by the National Autistic Society said that anxiety made it hard for them to get on with their lives.

Anxiety of this magnitude can result in exhaustion and breakdowns. It might also make autistic people tired and stressed out. A person's quality of life, including their physical and mental health, work and school life, and social life, can be significantly impacted by this.

You should seek additional guidance and support if you or someone you know is concerned about anxiety symptoms.

How can I get support and assistance?

Talking to your loved ones about what's worrying you might be helpful if anxiety is affecting your life. Discuss with your doctor if you feel you need more help.

Counseling, therapy, or medication may be offered by your primary care physician.

Therapy and counseling.
You can go to therapy or counseling privately or through your primary care physician. If properly adapted, a variety of therapies, including cognitive behavioral therapy (CBT), can be helpful for some autistic individuals.

Find information about counselors and therapists in your area who have experience working with autistic people in our Autism Services Directory.

Other strategies that may aid in stress and anxiety reduction include:

Ideally, all treatments should be administered by a professional who has a good understanding of autism. Examples of exposure therapy include working with a professional to gradually expose someone to the thing that makes them anxious. Low arousal techniques focus on stress reduction. sensory integration training helps with sensory differences. Most importantly, support should be tailored to a person's particular requirements in order to be effective and accessible.

Adult statutory guidance in England stipulates that autistic individuals with mental health issues should receive individualized support.

Medication You might be given medication, like a medication for depression. Although antidepressants are generally regarded as safe and effective, very little research has been conducted to determine whether they aid in the treatment of anxiety in autistic individuals. According to the available research, autistic individuals may be more likely to experience adverse effects like drowsiness, irritability, and decreased activity.

A medical professional should carefully consider and closely monitor antidepressants.

Advice and guidance The following is a list of some general advice and guidance from professionals and autistic individuals that you might want to try.

Keep a diary to keep track of the things that make you anxious and what might make it worse.

Keep an eye on your energy levels and take control of them. Keep an eye on your energy levels after social events and other difficult or exhausting activities. Take some time for yourself and do things you enjoy to recharge.

Make the environment work. Make adjustments whenever possible, such as dimming artificial lighting if it is too harsh.
To lessen sensory overload, try headphones that block out noise.

Self-soothe By using sensory tools and stimming, if that works for you, you can lower your anxiety levels.

Activities for calming and relaxation Try activities like yoga, meditation, mindfulness, and exercise for relaxation.

Visual schedules: Using visual schedules, you can organize your day and reduce uncertainty.

Utilize an app The following apps provide individualized anxiety support.

Brain in Hand consists of:
a system to monitor anxiety levels, individual coping strategies, and access to support from the National Autistic Society are all included in a diary.
Molehill Mountain consists of:

evidence-based advice on how to manage anxiety levels at home is provided by a system that keeps track of mood and identifies triggers. Children with autism experience many of the same anxieties and worries as other children.

However, things that normally developing children find less concerning may cause anxiety or worry in autistic children. Examples of these are:

Small disruptions to their routines or new body sensations, as well as social situations where it's hard to know what other people are thinking or feeling, particularly when it comes to physical symptoms that are unfamiliar or unpleasant and are linked to worried thoughts and feelings.

A child's anxiety may be reduced, but the behavior that is associated with the fundamental characteristics of autism will not disappear.

Anxiety symptoms in autistic children and adolescents When autistic children experience anxiety, their behavior may resemble typical autism features such as stimming, obsessive and ritualistic behavior, and resistance to changes in routine.

Additionally, autistic children are unable to always express their anxiety because they struggle to recognize their own anxious thoughts and feelings. You might, on the other hand, observe an increase in challenging behavior.

Your anxious child might, for instance:
Rely more on obsessions and rituals, like lining up or spinning objects, stim by rocking, spinning, or flapping hands, and do things to hurt themselves, like head-banging, scratching skin, or hand-biting, have more trouble sleeping, have meltdowns, emotional outbursts, and avoid or withdraw from social situations.

Anxiety is a normal part of life that everyone goes through at some point. However, there are some things you can do to alleviate your child's worries and help them control their own anxiety.

What causes anxiety?

How to spot them in autistic children and teens Identifying the factors that cause your autistic child to be anxious is the first step in easing their anxiety and assisting them in coping with it.

You may need to read your child's signals and figure out what makes your child feel anxious or stressed because autistic children and teens can have trouble understanding and managing their emotions.

Among the most common causes of anxiety in autistic children are:

changes in routine, such as missing a weekly piano lesson because the teacher is ill, changes in the environment, such as a new house, new play equipment at the local park, or furniture in different places at home. New social situations, such as a birthday party at an unfamiliar house. Sensory sensitivities, such as sensitivity to particular noises, bright lights, particular flavors or food textures. Fear of a specific situation, activity, or object, such as sleeping in their own bed, going to the bathroom, balloon
times of transition, such as the beginning of a new school year, secondary school, or puberty.
Making a list of the things that make your child feel anxious can help you figure out how to help him or her deal with these situations after you have identified some of the triggers.

Give your child numerous chances to practice handling these things and situations in secure settings.

It helps if the people who look after your child, like teachers, child care workers, and family members, also know what makes your child feel anxious and how they can help him or her deal with it.

Strategies for assisting autistic children in recognizing anxiety Your autistic child may need to understand how anxiety affects their body.

For instance, when your child experiences anxiety:
Their palms get sweat-soaked
they get a bizarre inclination in their stomach
their heart beats quicker
their hands fold.
You could try drawing a person's body in outline. Work with your child to draw or write on the outline what happens in each part of their body when they are afraid or worried.

Strategies for calming and relaxing autistic children when they start to feel anxious You can help your child learn how to relax when they start to feel anxious or stressed. Some examples might be:
Counting slowly to 10, taking five deep breaths, jumping 50 times on the trampoline, running around the yard, looking at a collection of special or favorite things, reading a favorite book, and closing your eyes for a few moments before going to a quiet area of the house. When your child is calm, encourage them to practice these techniques. You can gently encourage your child to try the strategies when they are anxious once they are well-versed in them.

Visual tools to help autistic children prepare for anxious situations If your child responds well to social stories and visual supports, you could use these tools to prepare for anxious situations.

You could, for instance, take pictures of your child doing things like walking through the school gate, sitting in the classroom, playing sports, eating lunch, and so on if your child gets anxious when you drop them off at school. You could also take pictures of the things you'll be doing apart, like driving home, going grocery shopping, gardening, etc. It would also be important to have a clear picture of you coming back to pick up your child.

Visual schedules on a daily or weekly basis can assist in preparing your child if they cause anxiety when there is a change in routine. You can indicate this on your schedule when you are aware of a change, such as swimming lessons will not be offered during the school holidays. Check the schedule with your child on a regular basis leading up to the change so that they are aware of how the weekly routine will change.

Some children prefer to be informed a day in advance of a change or event. Some prefer advance notification. However, for some, too much notice can cause them to worry until the event occurs.

Opportunities to practice in stressful or anxious situations Giving your child opportunities to practice in stressful situations can help them understand and feel more prepared for these situations.

Take your child for a practice run, for instance, if going to the hairdresser makes your child feel anxious. You could ask the hairdresser if you could come during the day when it is quiet and peaceful, and then you and your child could go through the steps together. Alternatively, your child might be able to observe another person cut their hair.

Assuming your kid gets restless in friendly circumstances you could rehearse these together. You could rehearse various circumstances and alternate assuming various parts. Encourage and praise your child while you try to keep the scenarios short and simple. Getting help managing anxiety in autistic children and teens A psychologist might be able to help if your child is extremely anxious. Psychologists can work directly with your child and family to develop strategies for reducing anxiety because they have specialized training in mental health conditions.

Psychologists employ a variety of methods, including:
The stepladder approach and other therapies and supports that use gradual exposure to help children face their fears, such as cognitive behavior therapy and social stories, can help prepare children for unfamiliar or stressful situations that typically make them anxious. Relaxation training can also assist your child in learning to relax. Your child may also benefit from the assistance of mental health occupational therapists in coping with anxiety.

You can ask your general practitioner or pediatrician to recommend a therapist or psychologist.

Children with autism may also benefit from medication to alleviate symptoms of anxiety. It is typically only recommended when behavior strategies have not sufficiently reduced a child's anxiety and it is affecting their daily life. This option can be discussed with your physician or pediatrician.

Anxiety levels among autistic children are higher than those of their peers. It is particularly challenging to accurately diagnose anxiety disorders and provide these children with effective treatment. Anxiety levels in autistic children may be linked to intellectual functioning, according to inconsistent evidence. The evidence is the subject of our first meta-analysis. 49 papers were identified for review after a systematic search. Anxiety and intelligence quotient tests were used in these papers on 18,430 autistic children. Correlation studies demonstrated a significant link between autistic children's intelligence quotient and anxiety: On anxiety tests, children with a higher intelligence quotient scored higher. This conclusion was also supported by studies directly comparing groups of autistic children with and without intellectual disabilities. This conclusion was also supported by the majority of studies with alternative designs. Utilizing a framework for quality assessment revealed typical threats to validity. A lot of studies used anxiety measures that were not consistent across the samples they were measuring. This was especially noticeable for children who were autistic and also had intellectual disabilities. Future studies need to figure out if the relationship between intelligence quotient and anxiety is indicative of something important in the mechanism that causes anxiety in autistic children or if our measures of anxiety lack sensitivity to different groups.

Lay abstract Autistic children frequently have higher anxiety levels than their peers. Due to the high degree of variability in their underlying abilities and presentations, it can be challenging to diagnose and treat anxiety disorders in autistic children. According to some evidence, autistic children who have a higher intelligence quotient (a measure of intelligence) are more likely to experience anxiety than autistic children who have a lower intelligence. However, other studies have not found a difference or found higher levels of anxiety in autistic children with lower intelligence, so the evidence is inconclusive. In order to determine whether autistic children with higher intelligence quotients experience more anxiety than autistic children with lower intelligence quotients, we conduct a literature review in this article. 49 papers on the subject were found through a methodical literature search. An objective framework for quality assessment was used to evaluate each paper's methods. There was statistical evidence that autistic children with higher intelligence quotients are more anxious than autistic children with lower intelligence quotients when the data were compared statistically. The quality review revealed common research flaws. Most importantly, only a small number of studies utilized anxiety scales that have been demonstrated to be reliable for children with very low intelligence quotients. In a similar vein, numerous studies utilized anxiety scales that have not been demonstrated to be appropriate for autistic children. Because children with autism and those with a low intelligence quotient may experience or comprehend anxiety in different ways, these factors are crucial. To determine whether autistic children's high intelligence quotient is linked to high levels of anxiety, future research should employ fully validated measures.

Keywords: anxiety, autism, autism spectrum disorder, intelligence quotient, and meta-analysis Autism is characterized by restricted or repetitive behaviors and interests as well as difficulties in social communication and interaction across multiple contexts (American Psychiatric Association, 2013). In the United Kingdom and the United States, approximately one to two percent of children are autistic, and diagnosis rates are rising annually (Baio et al., 2018; Russell and other, 2014). People with autism have different characteristics, and their symptoms frequently co-occur with those of other neurodevelopmental or psychiatric disorders (de Bruin et al., 2007; Leyfer et al., 2006). Anxiety disorders are among the most prevalent comorbidities (de Bruin et al., 2007; Lai et al. 2019; Mattila and team, 2010). According to the American Psychiatric Association (2013), anxiety disorders are a group of related conditions characterized by an emotional experience of anxiety coupled with excessive worry. Anxiety disorders frequently result in behavioral changes as well as physical symptoms, such as avoidance, difficulty sleeping, and muscle tension (American Psychiatric Association, 2013).

Anxiety in autistic children About 40% meet the criteria for an anxiety diagnosis (Mattila et al., 2010; Simonoff and other, White et al., 2008), with estimates ranging from 11 percent to 84 percent 2009), as opposed to between 2 and 24 percent of the general population (Merikangas et al., 2009). According to van Steensel et al., autistic children are twice as likely as their neurotypical peers to be diagnosed with an anxiety disorder. 2011). According to the American Psychiatric Association (2013), the trajectories of anxiety disorders in autistic children are comparable to those of children with anxiety disorders on their own. They typically begin as externalizing behaviors in younger children and progress to withdrawal and avoidance in adolescence. 2012, Kerns and Kendall; White and Co., 2009). However, sensory sensitivities are linked to more compulsions, social avoidance, and anxieties in autistic children (Acker et al., 2018). It is essential to understand anxiety in autistic children because having an anxiety disorder in addition to being autistic is associated with increased self-harm, depression, and parental stress in comparison to autism alone (Kerns et al., 2015) and diminished well-being (van Steensel et al., 2012). Additionally, there is a lot of evidence that autism research is a priority for the autism community (James Lind Alliance, 2016; Pellicano and others, 2014).

Anxiety, autism, and intellectual functioning The intellectual functioning of autistic children varies significantly (Charman et al., 2011). Half of autistic children have IQs above or below the normal range, but half also have a comorbid intellectual disability (ID; Charman and others, 2011), for which the diagnostic criteria call for an IQ below 70. According to Mattson & Shoemaker (2009), there is evidence that autistic children with the lowest IQ (those with comorbid ID) exhibit a distinct phenotype of autism, including an increased risk of challenging behavior and decreased adaptive behavior. Therefore, it is crucial to consider whether autistic children's intellectual functioning can predict other difficulties.

Contradictory findings exist, but there is some evidence that anxiety in autistic children varies with IQ. Anxiety disorders in autistic children have been linked to high IQ (Salazar et al., 2015). In contrast, other studies (Rosenberg et al.,) have found that low IQ may be linked to increased anxiety problems in autistic children. 2011; van Steensel and others, 2011). According to a recent meta-analysis (van Steensel &

Heeman, 2017), the highest-IQ autistic children had the greatest anxiety differences from their peers. This article only synthesized comparative data and looked at studies that directly compared neurotypical children. In addition, it excluded papers containing IDs for children with comorbid conditions. There is still no synthesis of the evidence that autistic children's IQ and anxiety are related. However, research in this area faces significant obstacles.

Problems with studying anxiety in autism and groups with low intelligence (Wood & Gadow, 2010) Due to the high degree of symptom overlap between anxiety disorders and autism, there are few effective measures for anxiety in autistic children. According to White et al., there is a lack of consensus regarding best practice measures and little consistency in the way anxiety in autistic children is measured in the literature. 2009). Because of this, it is difficult to make a clinical diagnosis, and published studies show a lot of methodological variation. Additionally, autistic children have a high prevalence of alexithymia, or the inability to recognize and express emotions (around 55%; Kinnaird and others, 2019) may make it difficult to measure anxiety, but little research has been done in this area. Parent reports are used in the majority of studies on anxiety in autistic children. Depending on a child's ability to communicate their feelings to their caregiver, relying on a parent's report may be problematic. The Child Adolescent Symptom Inventory–Anxiety (CASI-Anx;) is one of the well-validated measurement tools for anxiety in autistic children despite these challenges. Sprafkin and others, 2002) and the Parent Report for the Spence Children's Anxiety Scale (SCAS-P; Jitlina and other, 2017).

When we take into account those autistic children who have an ID, there are additional issues with reliability. Psychiatric disorders like anxiety are frequently underdiagnosed in ID patients because anxiety diagnostic criteria and assessment methods heavily rely on self or parent reports of anxiety verbalization or communication (Bailey & Andrews, 2003; Matson and others, 1997). People with ID may not be able to verbally express their worries or label complex internal states like anxiety because of their limited communication abilities. Despite this, there are still estimates of a higher prevalence of anxiety in ID (Emerson & Hatton, 2007). The Strengths and Difficulties Questionnaire (SDQ), for example, has been shown to accurately measure anxiety in children with ID. 2005, Emerson).

There are significantly fewer appropriate measures of anxiety for autistic children with comorbid ID, making it challenging to measure anxiety in this population. Anxiety scales appear to have been developed for people with ID or modified for use in "high-functioning" autism. There is no established standard for measuring anxiety in autistic children with comorbid ID, and few people take into account the effects of both on anxiety. The Autism Comorbidity Interview, Present and Lifetime Version (ACI-PL;) is one measure that has adequate reliability and validity in a sample of autistic children with IQs ranging from 42 to 141. Leyfer et al., 2006), but not many people use this.

49 studies were included in our systematic review. According to a meta-analysis of correlational studies, autistic children with higher IQ scored higher on anxiety measures, though only a small portion of the variance in anxiety was explained. This effect was strongest in studies with ID children, but it was not significant in studies without ID children.

A less common method has been to compare anxiety levels among groups of autistic children with lower and higher IQs. There were only four studies available here, and the data were unclear. A statistically significant difference, or a small-to-medium effect size, was found in three studies that were statistically identical, indicating that autistic children without comorbid ID experienced higher levels of anxiety. White & Roberson-Nay's 2009 study significantly increased the overall level of heterogeneity. The effect estimate changed significantly when the group was removed, revealing a significant difference between the groups. The heterogeneity was reduced to excellent levels as the CIs narrowed. This study scored poorly on the quality framework and had a significantly smaller sample size than the other three. The effect estimate is probably more accurately reflected in analyses that do not include this study. Three of the four studies comparing IQ scores between groups with high and low anxiety found no discernible differences. Six of the 14 papers that took different approaches, and many of them used more than one method of analysis, found significant results that were consistent with higher levels of anxiety being associated with higher IQ (n = 4760). On the other hand, seven studies (n = 2746) found no relationship between IQ and anxiety, and one of the studies was particularly large (Rosenberg et al., 2011) found that autistic children with comorbid ID had higher rates of anxiety diagnoses.

In autism, how and why are anxiety and IQ linked?
The hypothesis that autistic children with a higher IQ have higher levels of anxiety than autistic children with a lower IQ is broadly supported by the findings of this review. There was a clear, albeit small, positive correlation for studies involving children with IQs across

the board. In a similar vein, groups of autistic children who had ID displayed lower levels of anxiety than those who did not. There was no consistent evidence of a correlation between IQ and anxiety in studies that only included children with IQs in the normal range or higher. There are a number of plausible explanations for why there was a different pattern across these studies based on the current evidence. The existence of a linear relationship between IQ and anxiety across the entire range of IQs is one possibility. Testing across a narrower range of IQs would reveal smaller anxiety differences, necessitating greater statistical power to determine the effect. A previous meta-analysis (van Steensel & Heeman, 2017) that only looked at children with IQs in the normal range found that the children with the highest IQs had the greatest anxiety differences from their peers. A second possibility is that the correlation is supported by a non-linear relationship, in which case the large differences between people with IQs in the normal range and those with the lowest IQs are what cause the overall effect to be small. The group-level data lend some credence to this possibility. Last but not least, studies that excluded people with ID may have shared common methodological constraints due to methodological differences. These alternatives cannot be distinguished from the existing literature, so additional research—perhaps including a reanalysis of existing data sets—is crucial.

The reviewed papers suggested a variety of possible reasons why autistic children's IQ and anxiety are linked. According to some authors, this connection is directly related to the cognitive abilities associated with high IQ. According to Kerns & Kendall (2012), a high IQ allows for more abstract thinking and planning, which may increase the likelihood of anticipatory worries and associated anxiety.

Additionally, children with higher IQs may be better able to perform higher-order functions, which may make it easier for them to worry about the past, the future, or their own self-efficacy, which may make anxiety worse (Salazar et al., 2015). However, this pattern does not appear to apply to children who do not have autism (Karpinski et al., 2018; Martin and others, 2010; Penney and other, 2015). Higher IQ may interact with autistic children's social and functional experiences and expectations, according to alternative explanations. A higher IQ may lead to greater exposure to a wider variety of social settings and environments, such as mainstream education. These expose you to more situations that cause anxiety (Salazar et al., 2015). On the other hand, autistic children who have higher IQs may be better able to identify the gap between their social skills and those of their peers, which may lead to anxiety (Acker et al., 2018).

However, rather than differences in experience, the degree of measurement sensitivity may be to blame for these findings. It is difficult to assess anxiety in autistic children because many anxiety-related behavioral signs frequently overlap with autism symptoms (Wood & Gadow, 2010). According to Bailey & Andrews (2003), doing so with people who have lower IQs adds additional difficulty. This is in part because anxiety-related behavioral symptoms frequently overlap with undiagnosed health conditions in ID. Up to 73% of autistic children with comorbid ID suffer from gastrointestinal disorders, which frequently cause trouble sleeping, aggression, and self-injurious behavior (Mannion & Leader, 2016). According to Salazar et al., autistic children with higher IQs may be better at expressing their worries than autistic children with comorbid ID. 2015). Rarely are anxiety scales adapted for use with ID children who are autistic. These measures typically rely on anxiety reports from parents and on a child's capacity to label and communicate their feelings to a caregiver. Alternately, according to Bailey & Andrews (2003), these measures may require parents to observe anxiety-related behaviors, which frequently differ qualitatively in children with ID.

Because it has important clinical implications, it should be a top priority for research in the area to distinguish between these broad alternatives. More research is needed to determine how anxiety affects functioning and quality of life in autistic children with high IQs if this is the case. Children who are autistic and have higher IQs are more likely to have clinical anxiety, but they also likely have better ways of coping with anxiety. A greater focus on anxiety in autistic children with higher IQs would be supported by higher levels of anxiety and its associated impact on quality of life. The opposite is true if the observed differences indicate measurement sensitivity; In order to improve assessment, individuals with lower IQs require additional resources. In either case, current service providers and policymakers ought to exercise moderation. The current estimate suggests that the IQ of autistic children only accounts for a small portion of the variance in anxiety. Methodological limitations need to be addressed.

This is the first meta-analytic review of this research question in comparison to other reviews. It offers a fascinating point of comparison to a recent study on adults with autism. Hollocks and co. 2019) conducted a meta-analysis to determine whether having comorbid ID had any effect on autistic adult prevalence rates of anxiety and depression. They discovered that studies with autistic adults and comorbid ID had lower estimates of anxiety prevalence than studies with autistic adults alone, but these findings were not significant. These findings broadly correspond to those we observe in autistic children. Van Steensel & Heeman (2017) conducted a second meta-analysis to determine whether autistic children had higher rates of anxiety than typically developing children. Anxiety disorders were found to be more common in autistic children than in children with typical development, and IQ moderated this effect. That is, the gap between the anxiety levels of autistic children and those of typically developing children grows larger with increasing IQ. The findings of van Steensel and Heeman (2017) back up the ones in this review and suggest that the mechanism underlying the connection between IQ and anxiety may be unique to autistic children. Notably, van Steensel and Heeman (2017) did not include children with ID, which means that less is known about the mechanism in this group (less than half of autistic children; Charman and others, 2011).

The literature was sufficient to complete two meta-analyses that were methodologically sound, and additional papers provided narrative reports. It still has significant limitations. The heterogeneity of the literature (I2 = 81% and 77%) is one of the limitations of this review. Notably, removing a single study significantly reduced this in each case. Why this study was included in the meta-analysis of correlations (Niditch et al., 2012) reported such differences, suggesting that they may be specific to the population that was used. This was probably due to the small sample size and poor methodological quality of the group-level meta-analysis (White & Roberson-Nay, 2009).

Measures of anxiety accounted for the most methodological variation among the papers because there is no universally accepted method for evaluating anxiety in autistic children with comorbid ID. As a result, it's not clear whether anxiety measures used in different papers necessarily reflect the same concept.

Any meta-analysis's findings demonstrate the analytical strategy's ability to gather and extract data from returned search results. We decided to include papers wherever we could because of the small and diverse body of literature. One study was included, with participants ranging in age from 18 to 25 (Syriopoulou-Delli et al.,) with an average age of less than 18 years. 2019). The overall estimate was little affected by omitting this paper. Three author sets were unable to provide data for a paper that was returned by the search, and all of these papers reported a correlation that was not statistically significant (Johnson et al., 2015; 2004; Mayes and Calhoun Ozsivadjian and others, 2014). In this way, potential outcomes are a minimal over-distortion of genuine impact sizes.

The initial analytic decisions made by the authors of the returned papers frequently restrict meta-analytic processes. A linear relationship between IQ and anxiety was investigated in each of the 31 papers with correlations. Given that studies that excluded people with the lowest IQs did not identify an effect, our meta-analysis raises an important question regarding whether this was appropriate. Given the prevalent approach in the literature, it was essential to synthesize the data in this manner. Based on our data, it is clear that additional analytical methods should be considered in the future.

In addition to clarifying the nature of the relationship between IQ and anxiety in autistic children, future research is required to improve our methods of assessing and treating anxiety in this group. Clinical implications In particular, the development of anxiety tests for autistic children that are compatible with those with comorbid ID should be the primary focus of future research. The quality scoring revealed that this was a particularly weak area of the papers in this review, with the methods chosen frequently being inappropriate for use in autism and ID. Not only will having a gold standard for measuring anxiety make it easier to compare studies and come to valid conclusions, but it would also be a useful clinical tool to help diagnose anxiety in these groups. The recently developed Anxiety Scale for Children – ASD's psychometric properties (Rodgers et al., 2016), and Scahill et al.'s Parent-Rated Anxiety Scale for ASD 2019) look promising, but validation of these measures in larger populations will require additional research. It is essential to determine the mechanism by which IQ affects anxiety in autistic children because only then can treatments that are tailored to specific needs, including IQ level, be provided. According to van Steensel & Bogels (2015), it is evident that anxiety disorder interventions can be easily modified and are effective for autistic children. However, treatment response in autistic children who have an ID is rarely investigated. Regardless of whether an autistic child has a comorbid ID, anxiety levels are high (Mayes, Calhoun, Murray, Ahuja, et al., 2011). In light of the fact that children with comorbid ID have not been included in the research to date, it is necessary to develop interventions for anxiety in autistic children that are suitable for them. According to van Steensel & Bogels (2015), the majority of research into treatments for anxiety in autism, such as modified CBT, has focused on children with higher intellectual abilities.

In Conclusion, The existing body of research demonstrates a significant connection between autistic children's high IQs and their high levels of anxiety. Existing strategies for estimating tension in mentally unbalanced bunches with comorbid ID are poor. There are few measures that are tailored to this group and frequently rely on verbal labeling of complex emotional states. To determine whether the relationship between IQ and anxiety in autistic children is primarily driven by experience or measurement, additional research is required.

Chapter five:

Apprehension for the future

What is in store for the future?

When a child is given the diagnosis of autism spectrum disorder, one of the most common questions from parents is about their child's future. Will they be able to survive on their own? Will you wed? Did you go to school? Got a job? Sadly, psychologists cannot predict the future and frequently receive unsatisfactory responses to these crucial questions. However, we do know that there are a few factors that have been shown to predict children with autism spectrum disorder's long-term outcomes.

One of the most common concerns we hear from parents is worries about the future. Fortunately, we can rely on a few predictors to provide some insight into potential outcomes. Keep in mind that the term "predictors" does not imply a specific outcome!

The child's capacity to engage in independent living skills is one of these predictors. These skills are frequently taught more explicitly to children on the autism spectrum than to other children. As professionals and parents concentrate on academics or other skills, this is an essential aspect that is frequently overlooked, particularly for children with higher functioning abilities. However, research reveals that adaptive functioning skills deficits frequently exist regardless of cognitive functioning level. I believe it would be beneficial to review strategies for increasing independence given the significance of focusing on the development of skills necessary for daily living.

Plan Before you start, it can be helpful to make a plan. Make a list of skills for living on one's own that may be more challenging for your child but that other children his or her age frequently possess. Use this list as a guide rather than letting it overwhelm you. Concentrate only on a few skills at a time.

Utilization of Visual Supports Language comprehension is one obstacle to skill development. Children cannot fully benefit from their parents' instruction if they do not comprehend what is said to them.

Therefore, it is essential to use visual supports to complement verbal communication in these circumstances. A visual schedule is one kind of visual support that can be especially helpful. In this instance, a child is shown the various steps necessary to complete a skill through a visual schedule. When teaching a child to brush their teeth, for instance, you might break the process down into steps like picking up the toothbrush, applying toothpaste to it, wetting the toothbrush, brushing the top and bottom teeth, spitting, rinsing their mouth, rinsing the brush, and putting the toothbrush away. The next step is to point to each step as you complete it as you practice this skill with them. The child will be able to use the visual supports to complete the task more independently as a result of this improved understanding of the steps.

Shaping, Behaviors Gradually It is important not to expect a child to learn or start using a new skill right away. Changes in behavior that last a lifetime and the development of new skills take time. We must, instead, gradually alter behavior. This means that we need to set goals that are higher than the person's current level of functioning. Then, we emphasize achieving these objectives. The individual can gradually increase the goal if they achieve it more than 80% of the time. If we initially set the goal too high, the person is more likely to give up and become overly frustrated. If we set the goal too low, it's too easy, and we don't see any more progress. For determining progress and when to increase demands, it is very important to keep track of the frequency with which goals are met.

Addressing Other Skill Deficits or Sensory Sensitivities When teaching daily living skills, it is frequently apparent that a child may be unable to learn and use the skill due to other skill deficits or sensory sensitivities.

It's important to think about other treatments that might be needed. For instance, some children have difficulty dressing themselves on their own because they lack the fine motor skills to zip or button clothes. Due to sensory sensitivities, children may also refuse to take a bath or shower or brush their teeth. In order to treat these symptoms, these children probably would benefit from occupational therapy services.

Utilization of Positive Reinforcement When a skill or behavior is rewarded, it will occur more frequently. Therefore, it is essential to reinforce any progress made by a child when teaching them a new skill. The child may receive reinforcing privileges or praise (especially labeled praise, in which you name the behavior that pleases you), among other forms of reinforcement. When used consistently and as close to the behavior as possible, reinforcement is most effective.

Increasing Generalization It is essential to practice skills in a variety of settings in order to improve their generalizability. When starting out, it's often best to practice in a familiar setting. However, once your child has mastered the skill in that setting, it should be practiced in other, less familiar settings to help him or her adapt to new situations.

Your autistic child's future is unknown to anyone. When they are three, they won't be the same person at 13 or 30. Your child's development is not finished just because of an autism diagnosis!)

I ask people who join my Embracing Autism community what their biggest autism-related question is. In addition, my administrators and I have been hearing the same refrain more and more: "I just want my child to have the best future possible. "I wish I had known what would happen when my child gets older." "I just wish to help my child have a successful and healthy life in the future." It is so transparent that parents or guardians are seriously concerned about the future of their autistic children, and I do not blame them for this.

You see, doctors can give you a lot of anxiety when they give your child an autism diagnosis.

Your child will never communicate because they are nonverbal.

Your child may never be capable of living on their own or pass out from high school.

Your child won't be able to make friends easily and may never have any real relationships.

Sound familiar?

However, I'm going to tell you a little secret today... It all comes down to this:

3 Isn't 13. 13 is not 30.

You have to understand that your child today is not the same person they will be in ten or twenty years.

And no one, not even your child's therapists or doctors, knows what the future holds for your autistic child.

Take a deep breath if your child has trouble communicating, developing social skills, or having meltdowns. because just because they struggled with a problem as children doesn't mean they'll always struggle with the same issues.

Take a look at it. What were some of your challenges in elementary school?

I'd bet that you don't still engage in those same actions.

When an autism diagnosis is given to a child, many parents mistakenly believe that their child's life and development have come to an end.

But the fact of the matter is that your child is constantly developing in new ways and learning new things.

My son used to only talk to movie scripts when he got the diagnosis, but now he talks to everyone.

And a disclaimer: We simply followed his lead, connected with him, and supported him in his own natural development timeline, not by putting him through hours and hours of intensive autism therapies.

Also, my son was diagnosed when he was 4 and is now 8 years old. Imagine what he will be doing when he is 14 years old!

The fact of the matter is that no one knows the future of your autistic child at this time.

None of the medical professionals, therapists, or even me.

Although I am able to state that my son has made significant progress in his development since we became aware of his diagnosis and gained a better understanding of how to provide him with support, I am also able to acknowledge that some autistic children will continue to be non-speakers well into adulthood.

But here is the problem: It is acceptable that your autistic child will not speak into adulthood!

Numerous adult autistics who do not speak are living wonderful lives.

Even though these autistic people are still unable to speak, have meltdowns, or struggle with social situations, they are still very different people from when they were children.

See, an autistic person is still developing even though their autistic behaviors do not change.

Even though it is challenging for others to observe and comprehend that development, all autistic people are simply developing on their own natural timeline.

Don't make assumptions about your child based on their diagnosis. The main point of this post is this: Your autistic child's identity at age 3 does not predict who they will be at 13 or 30.

Therefore, I would like to put you to the test: Don't restrict your child based on their abilities when they are diagnosed.

Keep in mind that even after receiving their diagnosis, your autistic child will continue to grow and develop in their own unique way.

When a baby is six months old, no one says, "They can't talk, so clearly they won't ever talk" or "They can't walk, clearly they won't walk on their own."

With autistic children, it's much better to assume competence.

Make the assumption that your child will be able to carry out any task they choose. Make the assumption that your child is capable of learning and growing at their own pace.

Then, as their parent, your job is to assist your child as much as possible in that development.

I swear, from there, everything becomes a whole lot simpler!

The spectrum of autism (ASD) is extremely diverse. ASD sufferers may exhibit contradictory symptoms. Some ASD kids don't like to be squeezed and can't even stand a handshake. Other kids want the feeling so much they bump into other people's bodies. People sometimes don't immediately notice that people with ASD are different because they are so high functioning. They may also be unable to speak or meet their physical needs. ASD sufferers' futures can be as unpredictable as their symptoms. The future of people with ASD is determined by their strengths, interests, and skill sets, just like that of neurotypical people.

It's very important to have in mind that just because your kid has an ASD diagnosis doesn't mean they can't get to meet new people, date, go to college, get married, have to bear children, or have a fulfilling and successful career. Children with ASD need the same skills that normally developing children do in order to be successful adults; But it's important to remember that this process often looks different from how a typical child experiences things as they grow up to adulthood. At this point, it is common knowledge that children with ASD have better outcomes when they are diagnosed early and given evidence-based therapies to help them develop the skills they need to be successful children and adults. Applied behavioral analysis is the most effective and well-known treatment for helping individuals or children with ASD development and functional life skills. Children may also benefit from speech therapy, physical therapy, and occupational therapy, depending on their areas of growth.

Marriage and autism:

A person's diagnosis of ASD need not prevent them from getting married. People with ASD need partners who understand and respect their needs, just like in any relationship. Sometimes, they might need to communicate with partners in a more direct way, telling them exactly what they want and need rather than waiting for them to intuit it. This need not necessarily be restricted to couples in which one member has ASD. Every couple has to find a way to communicate that works for them. Adults with ASD who are struggling to navigate a romantic relationship can frequently benefit from the guidance of an experienced couples therapist. In fact, ASD is not the focus of the techniques used in couples therapy, which already emphasize teaching couples to take turns talking and making sure they understand each other.

Autism and Careers: What a person with ASD can do in a career depends on their skills. Naturally, this also applies to the general population. Several ASD sufferers who have achieved great success have written about this.

Dr. Temple Grandin, who is probably the most well-known person with ASD today, has some great advice for choosing a career when you have ASD based on how you think:
Some advice for those with autism or Asperger's syndrome in the workplace:

Every job should have a clear objective or end point.
Focus on your work rather than your persona. Organize your work into a portfolio.
Your social limitations must be acknowledged by the boss.
High functioning autistics and people with Asperger's syndrome should choose a college major in a field where they can find work. Because many of the best programmers probably have Asperger's syndrome or some of its symptoms, computer science is a good choice. Other great majors include: engineering, accounting, art, and library science, with a focus on commercial art and drafting. Avoid majors in English, political science, history, business, or pure mathematics. However, a major in library science can be combined with a minor in history; however, a degree in library science makes it easier to land a good job.

Encouragement should be given to some students to enroll in drafting, computer programming, or commercial art courses at a nearby college while they are still in high school. This will keep them motivated and protect them from being teased. How can low-income families afford computers for their children to learn programming or computer-aided drafting? When a business or engineering firm upgrades their equipment, used computers can frequently be obtained for free or at a very low cost. Many people are unaware that schools, banks, factories, and other businesses keep a lot of usable older computers in their storage areas. Although it won't be the most cutting-edge innovation, it will be sufficient for a student to learn on.

Final thoughts: A person with Asperger's syndrome or autism must overcome their lack of social skills by excelling in a specialized field to the point where others are willing to "buy" their skill, despite their lack of social skills. It's crucial to keep a portfolio of your work because of this. You will need to acquire some social survival skills, but if you share your interests with others who work in your field, you will make friends at work. The majority of my social life is devoted to my job. People I work with on interesting projects are friends of mine.

Dr. Grandin was successful in securing a job that allowed her to pursue her unusual way of thinking and her passion. She has revolutionized the way slaughterhouses operate today, humanizing and speeding up the process in ways that a neurotypical individual probably could not have imagined.

In addition to being a highly successful author, John Elder Robinson was able to use his "aspergian strengths" in a career in technology. Most notably, he constructed the "kiss" band's trick guitars. His autobiography, "Look Me in the Eye," is a great window into his unique way of thinking and provides a clear picture of a functioning adult with autism spectrum disorder.

Chapter six:
Myths and facts about autism

A developmental disability known as autism spectrum disorder (ASD) has symptoms that vary widely from person to person. Adults with ASD may learn, interact with others, and navigate the world in different ways.

Even though autistic people make up more than 2% of the population, many people have misconceptions about the condition. Experts have been working to dispel misunderstandings about the disability so that we can better comprehend the difficulties that ASD sufferers face.

Myth: Autism usually doesn't affect girls.
According to clinical psychologist Catherine Lord, PhD, who focuses on autism at the David Geffen School of Medicine at UCLA, girls are less likely to be diagnosed with autism. When compared to girls, boys are four times more likely to be diagnosed with ASD. While boys are still more likely to be born with ASD, it is also true that girls are more likely to be misdiagnosed when they do have it.

Additionally, ASD can run in families. Lord asserts that there is a genetic component. If you have an ASD-positive sibling or even a second-generation relative like an aunt or cousin, for instance, you are more likely to be diagnosed. According to Lord, children whose fathers are of older paternal age also have a slightly higher risk of being diagnosed with ASD.

Myth: ASD affects everyone in a similar way.

A wide range of experiences and symptoms characterize people with autism. Autism Speaks' Arianna Esposito points out that the challenges, behaviors, and skill sets of people with ASD can vary greatly from person to person. Because ASD encompasses a wide range of conditions, every person's experience with autism is unique, she asserts.

According to Esposito, ASD causes brain differences that are not well understood, and symptoms can vary significantly from person to person. Due to the wide range of symptoms, no two people have the same life experiences. She states, "If you only know one person with ASD, that really means you only know one person with such a condition."

In the Diagnostic and Statistical Manual of Mental Disorders 5 (DSM-5), autism was given the new name of autism spectrum disorder (ASD) in 2013. In order to include people with disabilities of varying degrees, the new name was chosen.

Myth: The majority of ASD suffer from severe intellectual disabilities.

No. According to Lord, the majority of people with ASD in the United States do not have severe intellectual disabilities and are able to function fairly normally in society. However, this is not the case globally. People with ASD almost exclusively have intellectual disabilities in nations like India that lack specialized support systems and are less likely to diagnose it except in extreme cases.

It is also a myth that the majority of people on the autism spectrum possess remarkable abilities like photographic memory or prodigal musical abilities. It happens, but it doesn't happen often, Lord says in Myth: Autism is caused by vaccines.

According to Esposito, there is absolutely no evidence that any vaccinations increase the risk of ASD.

Myth: More children are developing autism as a result of factors in the environment.

It is now more common to diagnose autism. In the United States, ASD affects one in 44 children, up from one in 88 a decade ago, according to the CDC. However, it is unlikely that the increase is environmental.

Lord asserts that a few factors are supported by the majority of the evidence. First, the way we describe children with autism has changed, and the disability now encompasses a variety of conditions, including Asperger's syndrome, autism disorder, and pervasive developmental disorder. The likelihood of a diagnosis has also increased as a result of increased awareness of the condition. The majority of the increase is probably due to these two factors.

Myth: Only when you were a child can you be diagnosed.

No. In point of fact, as our comprehension of the condition advances, an increasing number of adults are receiving autism diagnoses. Lord explains that this is because, in contrast to conditions like high blood pressure, ASD cannot be diagnosed using a biological marker. Because doctors don't realize that ASD is the underlying cause of their symptoms, many people are misdiagnosed as children with conditions like ADHD and anxiety.

Lord adds that her research has demonstrated that some individuals may fit into the category of ASD, but that as they get older, their symptoms become more pronounced due to the circumstances of their lives.

Facts

Autism in Adulthood

There are a number of reasons why people with autism may not be diagnosed until they are adults.

Autism doesn't just affect kids; it also affects adults as well.

Autism isolates autistic people and their families, which can lead to mental health issues.

In the United Kingdom, only 16% of adults with autism are employed full-time.

Support and intervention can significantly enhance the adult with autism's quality of life, despite the fact that the condition cannot be cured.

One in three adults with autism suffers from severe mental health issues in their lifetime as a result of a lack of support.

Many adults who would be considered to have autism were never given a diagnosis because the definition of autism changes.

Work-related activities that encourage independence have been shown in studies to improve daily living skills and reduce autism symptoms.

Surprising Information About Autism The word "autism" comes from the Greek word "autos," which means "self." The literal translation is "alone."

A child with autism can be diagnosed before he or she is 18 months old.

Not all people with autism are savants or nonverbal. It's a disorder on the spectrum.

Boys are diagnosed with autism more than four times more frequently than girls are.

People with autism have feelings, despite the fact that they may appear to be indifferent. a lot of emotions that can sometimes be overwhelming.

Autism increases the likelihood of other health problems, such as epilepsy, anxiety, and ADHD, in children.

Positive Autism Facts: Children with autism are extremely imaginative.

Autism sufferers excel at paying attention to the smallest of details and are thorough and accurate, which is advantageous in occupations like quality control that require this skill.

Visual learners are more common in autistic people.

On the spectrum, people are brutally honest, loyal, and dedicated to their work.

People with autism are able to become experts in their fields thanks to their extensive knowledge.

Autism patients are less likely to judge other people. They are very open to differences.

People with autism are resilient and determined.

Some autistic people may experience feelings of isolation and loneliness as a result of misconceptions. In extreme cases, it may also result in bullying and abuse.

There are numerous misconceptions and myths associated with autism spectrum disorder.
From "refrigerator mothers" to the idea that everyone with autism is like "Rain Man," this disorder has been widely misunderstood in the past.

Furthermore, numerous misconceptions and myths persist today.
The top five myths as we see them, along with an explanation of the actual truth, are listed below!

Myth: Vaccination causes autism. Despite numerous large-scale, gold-standard scientific studies, there is simply no scientific evidence to support this.

We would already know if it were that straightforward. Chemical imbalance is complicated and is by all accounts brought about by various mixes of qualities and natural impacts. The promise of a quick and simple solution, a sudden stop to autism, or even a quick cure, has lured many parents.

Life isn't always easy, but you can be sure that a lot of work is being done to figure out the genes and other factors so that we can better understand autism and treat its symptoms.

Myth: individuals or Children with autism don't wish to make friends. This is almost never the case. There are some adults and children who are extremely distant from others and prefer to avoid them to a great extent. However, most people on the spectrum, both children and adults, enjoy socializing.

The problem with our children is that they frequently make mistakes and do not know how to interact with others. Being social is like dancing, which requires quick thinking and a lot of complex steps. It may seem too difficult. However, our children can learn by slowing down the dance and explaining the steps.

People on the spectrum may experience severe social anxiety, particularly if they have previously failed. However, the desire to connect is frequently present, and it is the responsibility of our loved ones' families, teachers, and therapists to facilitate social interaction.

Myth: Children with autism cannot learn. They can, provided that we as adults learn to teach them effectively. The vast majority of children will benefit from therapy, but it must be individualized and effective.

Learning can be challenging for some people, and their progress will be sluggish.

But things can change and people's lives can get better slowly and steadily as long as family and teachers keep trying and use a good teaching method.

Myth: Bad parenting is the root of autism. Sorry, but that simply isn't the case. Any child will not benefit from bad parenting, and neither will autism.

Because our children are not responding to us in the manner that a typical child would, many of us parents believe that we are not doing a good enough job of being parents. If we have multiple children but only one of them is on the spectrum, this is crystal clear.

However, we can raise each of our children to be excellent parents. Furthermore, the better we comprehend our youngsters, the more they can thrive.

Myth: People with autism, like Rain Man, have savant skills. Not everyone can recite the phone book or tell someone when they were born what day of the week it was. Absolutely certain individuals can do some astounding memory accomplishments, yet this isn't normal.

Some of the strengths that many children on the spectrum share are visual learners and good visual memory. Children can use these strengths to navigate the world.

Science versus pseudoscience When your child is first diagnosed with autism, it can be extremely difficult to accept the news. Your child's future may be uncertain, and the road ahead may appear daunting.

Right now a few guardians might go looking for a 'convenient solution' or remedy for their kid's chemical imbalance (read more about relieving mental imbalance), which makes them defenseless against pseudoscientific medicines.

What, then, is pseudoscience? It is described as "anything at all that pretends to be science that's not by any means" by Wikipedia. To put it simply, it is "fake science."

When a theory or idea is taken and an experiment is designed to rigorously test whether or not that theory is correct, that is good science.

A controlled clinical trial is one way we can accomplish this. In a controlled trial, the intervention we are testing, such as a new therapy, is compared to another treatment or no treatment in two closely matched groups, such as two autism-prone preschoolers.

Since the therapy is the only thing that differs between the two groups in a well-designed trial, we can reasonably assume that the therapy is having an effect if positive changes only occur in the therapy group.

In order to ensure that the same outcomes are achieved, the trial should ideally be repeated at least once, preferably by a different group of researchers. Medicines that go through this kind of thorough testing are called 'proof based.'

Pseudoscientists use a lot of scientific language, and their theories can appear to be quite convincing at first. However, they have little interest in determining whether or not their "treatment" is effective. You might even hear them say that controlled trials are unnecessary.

Some autistic people may experience feelings of isolation and loneliness as a result of misconceptions. In severe cases, it may also turn out into bullying and abuse.

There are numerous misconceptions and myths associated with autism spectrum disorder.
From "refrigerator mothers" to the idea that everyone with autism is like "Rain Man," this disorder has been widely misunderstood in the past.

Furthermore, numerous misconceptions and myths persist today.
The top five myths as we see them, along with an explanation of the actual truth, are listed below!

Myth: Vaccination causes autism. Despite numerous large-scale, gold-standard scientific studies, there is simply no scientific evidence to support this.
We would already know if it were that straightforward. Chemical imbalance is complicated and is by all accounts brought about by

various mixes of qualities and natural impacts. The promise of a quick and simple solution, a sudden stop to autism, or even a quick cure, has lured many parents.

Life isn't always easy, but you can be sure that a lot of work is being done to figure out the genes and other factors so that we can better understand autism and treat its symptoms.

Myth: individuals or Children with autism don't want to make friends. This is almost never the case. There are some adults and children who are extremely distant from others and prefer to avoid them to a great extent. However, most people on the spectrum, both children and adults, enjoy socializing.

The problem with our children is that they frequently make mistakes and do not know how to interact with others. Being social is like dancing, which requires quick thinking and a lot of complex steps. It may seem too difficult. However, our children can learn by slowing down the dance and explaining the steps.

People on the spectrum may experience severe social anxiety, particularly if they have previously failed. However, the desire to connect is frequently present, and it is the responsibility of our loved ones' families, teachers, and therapists to facilitate social interaction.

Myth: Children with autism cannot learn. They can, provided that we as adults learn to teach them effectively. The vast majority of children will benefit from therapy, but it must be individualized and effective.

Learning can be challenging for some people, and their progress will be sluggish.

But things can change and people's lives can get better slowly and steadily as long as family and teachers keep trying and use a good teaching method.

Myth: Bad parenting is the root of autism. Sorry, but that simply isn't the case. Any child will not benefit from bad parenting, and neither will autism.

Because our children are not responding to us in the manner that a typical child would, many of us parents believe that we are not doing a good enough job of being parents. If we have multiple children but only one of them is on the spectrum, this is crystal clear.

However, we can raise each of our children to be excellent parents. Furthermore, the better we comprehend our youngsters, the more they can thrive.

Myth: People with autism, like Rain Man, have savant skills. Not everyone can recite the phone book or tell someone when they were born what day of the week it was. Absolutely certain individuals can do some astounding memory accomplishments, yet this isn't normal.

Some of the strengths that many children on the spectrum share are visual learners and good visual memory. Children can use these strengths to navigate the world.

Science versus pseudoscience When your child is first diagnosed with autism, it can be extremely difficult to accept the news. Your child's future may be uncertain, and the road ahead may appear daunting.

Right now a few guardians might go looking for a 'convenient solution' or remedy for their kid's chemical imbalance (read more about relieving mental imbalance), which makes them defenseless against pseudoscientific medicines.

What, then, is pseudoscience? It is described as "anything that pretends to be science but is not at all" by Wikipedia. To put it simply, it is "fake science."

When a theory or idea is taken and an experiment is designed to rigorously test whether or not that theory is correct, that is good science.

A controlled clinical trial is one way we can accomplish this. In a controlled trial, the intervention we are testing, such as a new therapy, is compared to another treatment or no treatment in two closely matched groups, such as two autism-prone preschoolers.

Since the therapy is the only thing that differs between the two groups in a well-designed trial, we can reasonably assume that the therapy is having an effect if positive changes only occur in the therapy group.

In order to ensure that the same outcomes are achieved, the trial should ideally be repeated at least once, preferably by a different group of researchers. Medicines that go through this kind of thorough testing are called 'proof based.'

Pseudoscientists use a lot of scientific language, and their theories can appear to be quite convincing at first. However, they have little interest in determining whether or not their "treatment" is effective. You might even hear them say that controlled trials are unnecessary.

CONCLUSION

Despite the fact that it is a prevalent issue in society, autism is a disorder that science has not yet thoroughly investigated. Therapists have only a limited understanding of how to diagnose it, comprehend its causes, and evaluate its impact on human life. Despite the fact that autism is a disease that has received little research, scientists now have the information they need to modify and control how it affects a person and reduce its adult manifestations.

Autism is a broad term for social perception because it encompasses a variety of different abnormalities that are linked to a person's behavioral characteristics. From a scientific standpoint, it is correct to refer to this condition as an autism spectrum disorder (ASD) because scientists classify various ASDs according to their symptoms and severity. However, according to Lord, Elsabbagh, Baird, & Veenstra-Vanderweele (2018), autism is typically characterized by a lack of social communication and recurrent sensory-motor behaviors that are caused by genetic or other factors. Even though society often thinks of autism as a disease that affects a person's intellectual abilities, this definition shows that autism is a disorder that affects social functions. On the other hand, people with autism exhibit exceptional intellectual abilities in certain fields, such as mathematics, art, or history.

If their external symptoms of the disorder are mild, autistic people can today get a higher education, get a job, have a family, and live like normal people in society. However, if autism has a higher degree of manifestation, they may also struggle with social communication, public spaces, and even daily routine. Even if an intellectual ability is highly developed, a person with a problem with sensory perception can be scared by loud noises or crowds. Additionally, people with autism may experience cramps, speech disorders, or limb recurrences that make it difficult for them to live independently. However, with the right treatment and development of social and commutative skills, autistic individuals typically become full members of society.

Both worldwide and in the United States, the number of people with autism disorders has increased in recent years (Sealeya et al., 2016). However, there may be a correlation between this trend and a rise in the accuracy of child disorder diagnoses and early detection. For instance, Kitzerow, Teufel, Wilker, and Freitag (2015) state that the short-term observation of change in social communication is a method that aids in the measurement of autism symptoms and produces observable results. Early intervention in the development of autism and the elimination of its external manifestations were made easier by this method of measuring and studying the condition. Because of this shift in evaluation and treatment methods, the intellectual and social development of people with autism can sometimes be as successful as that of people without the disorder. There are likewise alternate ways for deciding chemical imbalance that specialists generally use for finding, and they depend on side effects that manifest at various phases of an individual's life. These approaches differ depending on how much emphasis is placed on particular secular aspects of the individual's growth and interactions with the outside world.

Because they can manifest in a variety of ways based on the stage and characteristics of development, symptoms are conditionally divided into sensory, communicative, and social. The inability of a child or adult to maintain social connections, communicate with others, and recognize their emotions is an expression of social symptoms. Young children may avoid interacting with their parents and may not respond well to their names. Repetition of words and phrases, inability to concentrate on the subject at hand, and inability to respond to questions are all signs of communication problems in children. A weak or stronger response to light, sound, smell, and other external stimuli is associated with sensory symptoms. Another visible sign of the disorder is a pattern of gestures or actions that are repeated. By using these early indicators, parents and doctors can diagnose autism and stop it from getting worse.

However, despite extensive research into the symptoms of autism, scientists still struggle to identify the disorders' root causes. According to Lord et al., researchers have found a strong link between genetic causes and autism spectrum disorders. 2018). This statement indicates that an autism mutation can occur; However, this issue has not yet received sufficient research to establish a causal link between the disorder's occurrence and any genetic characteristics. Another study found that environmental factors like synthetic, neurochemical, and aromatic chemicals can affect the fetus and cause autism (Sealeya et al., 2016). Although there isn't yet a complete list of proven facts and data, environmental factors may play a role in autism. In addition, numerous studies demonstrate that there is no link between vaccines and autism, disproving the widespread misconception that vaccines cause the condition. Additionally, moral pressure and psychological trauma have been linked to developmental delays and autism symptoms (Sealeya et al., 2016). Because they cannot alter the underlying causes, the methods for preventing autism are constrained by the data's uncertainty.

However, some practices aid in the development of a person's social, communicative, and motor skills and reduce the impact of autism on daily life. Because young children are most susceptible to learning and therapy, autistic people need to be diagnosed as soon as possible for treatment to be effective. However, the process of developing abilities becomes more challenging as an adult. According to recent research (Robertson & Baron-Cohen, 2017), one of the most effective methods for early detection of autism is the identification of sensory symptoms. Medication to treat insomnia and convulsions, general therapy, and training to improve social and communication skills can all be part of the treatment process. Therapy also aims to get rid of fears and panic attacks caused by bright lights or loud noises. According to the findings of Bruin, Blom, Smit, Ja van Steensel, and Bögels (2015), mindfulness training improves the quality of life and social communication of autistic adolescents and their parents. An alternative that works well is also the use of other therapeutic interventions; However, they must take into account the unique characteristics of each autism disorder.

Problems with a person's social, communication, and sensory abilities are the hallmarks of autism. There is no link between this disorder and intellectual disability, and autistic people frequently have highly developed skills. Due to the lack of sufficient scientific investigation into the causes of this issue, there are few means of preventing it. However, there are numerous treatments and methods for managing autism symptoms that enable individuals with the condition to enhance their skills, participate in society, and lead normal lives.

The purpose of this final chapter was to provide a summary of the study as well as recommendations and conclusions based on all of the data presented in the preceding chapters. The goal was to provide a concise overview of the study's focus and outcomes.

The researcher is of the opinion that the results of this study will be beneficial to the social work field as a whole, and play therapy in particular. It offers a different approach to treating autistic children and a deeper comprehension of the autism phenomenon. This, it is accepted, will upgrade the chance of more suitable social way of behaving and in this manner give

support for the groups of mentally unbalanced people.

This research has required a lot of time and effort, but it has also provided a lot of enjoyment and satisfaction. It has been challenging because the focus area is one that many people, including the researcher, view as relatively new and unexplored. As a result, the researcher needed to learn a lot and understand a lot, which made him or her want to keep working with autistic children.

The researcher is currently treating autistic children through the use of play therapy at The Key School for Specialized Education in Parktown West. This is a direct result of this study and stems from the changes that were observed in the autistic children who participated in the play technique program. The researcher continues to recognize the advantages of play therapy, particularly with autistic children, and continues to derive numerous rewards from observing these children's improved social behavior.